The Positive Ageing Plan

The Positive Ageing Plan

The Expert Guide to Healthy, Beautiful Skin at Every Age

Dr Vicky Dondos

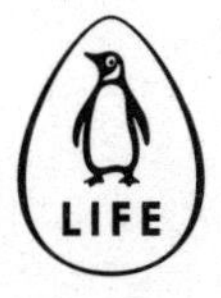

PENGUIN LIFE

AN IMPRINT OF

PENGUIN BOOKS

PENGUIN LIFE

UK | USA | Canada | Ireland | Australia
India | New Zealand | South Africa

Penguin Life is part of the Penguin Random House group of companies
whose addresses can be found at global.penguinrandomhouse.com.

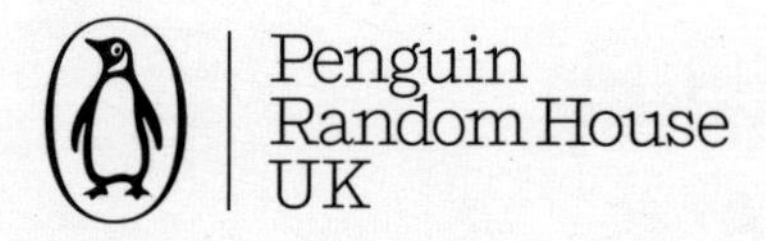

First published 2021
001

Set in 11/15pt Yoga Sans Pro
Typeset by Jouve (UK), Milton Keynes
Printed and bound in Great Britain by Clays Ltd, Elcograf S.p.A.

The authorized representative in the EEA is Penguin Random House Ireland, Morrison Chambers, 32 Nassau Street, Dublin D02 YH68

A CIP catalogue record for this book is available from the British Library

ISBN: 978-0-241-46424-3

www.greenpenguin.co.uk

Penguin Random House is committed to a sustainable future for our business, our readers and our planet. This book is made from Forest Stewardship Council® certified paper.

To my mother and father.
The driving force behind me, since day dot.

Contents

Prologue

Looking good feels good. At every age.

Here's the thing: you can be a woman with brains and gravitas and still spend time and money on maintaining and enjoying your appearance. Your appearance both communicates and influences your physical, mental, emotional and social wellbeing and it is *OK* to acknowledge its importance.

> 'It is not the desire to be beautiful that is wrong - but the obligation to be.'
>
> *A Woman's Beauty: A Put Down or Power Source*,
> by Susan Sontag (1975)

And it's OK to still care about your looks at 50, 60, 70 . . . In fact, I say it's important. Feeling beautiful transcends youth. And an attitude shift means we are finally catching up with our Parisian counterparts who have no 'use-by' date, no age limit to feeling and being attractive, and sexy: hallelujah!

But ageing is tough, even for those of us who try our hardest to focus on the positives and feel grateful. And to most women, what we see in our reflection matters. It can pull us down - or up - boosting our confidence, putting a spring in our step, sometimes turning our day around. Not to mention how feeling good about our appearance can be a powerful motivator to take steps to improve our general health. It's win, win.

So, let's start a new conversation about the role of 'beauty'. The approach I share in this book has come about as a culmination of my experiences as a doctor and co-founder of one of London's leading aesthetic medicine clinics for almost 15 years: I call it Positive Ageing. Which means reframing the way we understand and respond to changes in our body so that we can show ourselves the empathy and care we deserve. It's not about looking younger, but about looking and feeling good about yourself no matter your age.

When I started in aesthetics 15 years ago, you may be surprised but I was one of the very few female doctors working in this area. One of my first lines of research was to take myself off to appointments, to have my face examined and treatments recommended, at some of the biggest London clinics.

It's not that those clinics were bad, but they didn't make me feel part of the process, knowledgeable about health or good about myself. What I experienced made me realize that there needed to be a new way to treat women who had taken the big step to come into a clinic. And it had to be kinder, less critical, less judgemental and more holistic.

In this book I share the approach I developed, the Positive Ageing Pyramid (PAP). It gives you the frank inside scoop on everything you want to know about skincare, aesthetic treatments and the lifestyle habits and hacks that will enable you to understand and care for your health and appearance, in the best way that works for you. In this book:

1. I will demystify the ageing process, explain how it's intimately bound up with your health and what you can do to prevent premature ageing.
2. I will reveal my 5 basics of skincare that should be in everyone's routine, and list the products that are/aren't worth buying, and hopefully save your bank balance in the process.
3. I will explain the cosmetic treatment options available, what I think of them, who they're best for.
4. I will show you how to create **your own personalized programme**: how to look fresh, radiant, a 'best-version-of-me', at any age.

Knowing the facts will help you decide what you want to do, and how much time and money you want to spend doing it. Do you want to know how to prevent premature ageing, things like wrinkles or pigmentation? Do you want to know what all the fuss is about around certain products? Do you want to try and resolve an issue without having to see a doctor? Are you thinking of having more invasive treatment to tweak your appearance? Do you want to make your skin glow? (It's a yes to that one, right?!)

Whatever your reasons for being here, this is a science-based, straight-talking, judgement-free guide to finding the best options for your skin. In this book I explore everything proven to make a difference, from the basics to the more medical: exercise, sleep, food and digestion, skincare, suncare, and all the options when it comes to clinic treatments too.

I look at all the pros and cons for each one so that you have all the information to make your own decisions about what is best for you. You might want to dip into certain sections if there is something in particular you want to know; otherwise I recommend reading from the beginning, as the book is in chronological order according to the process I go through with my clients, and I really think this will make the most sense when you come to create your own plan.

The premise of the PAP is that building up your regime from the base of the pyramid will lead to the best outcome for your skin. I will refer to this throughout the book, as it is crucial to an effective, personalized plan at the end. Let me talk you through it.

PAP - Positive Ageing Pyramid

AESTHETIC MEDICINE

OPTIMIZE

REGENERATE

MAINTAIN

ACTIVE SKINCARE

LIFESTYLE MEDICINE

STRESS | NUTRITION | HORMONES | ENVIRONMENT

MINDSET

FEAR OF AGEING → NEGATIVE SELF-TALK → SELF-JUDGEMENT → BODY & APPEARANCE POSITIVITY

LEVEL 1: MINDSET This is the foundation. I cannot stress enough how important achieving a healthy mindset is before moving up the pyramid. This refers both to your approach to ageing and, even earlier in life, to the emotional component of what you see in the mirror. You can have the absolute best lifestyle, skincare, facials, and even injectables, but if your mind isn't in the right place, nothing will make you feel good.

For most people it takes just a little investigation to work out where their head is; for some people this takes some more self-reflection, but it is an essential step for everyone. We will look at the first three elements of the pyramid - fear of ageing, negative self-talk and self-judgement - in order to reach the final brick, appearance positivity.

LEVEL 2: LIFESTYLE This section contains the most up-to-date science on the lifestyle medicine that will support your skin. It's divided into four key areas - Stress, Nutrition and Digestion, Hormones and Environment - because these are the core areas, where the evidence shows that simple changes will result in visible change. For those of you who simply want to know how your genetics, diet, lifestyle and environment are really influencing your appearance, and what you can do to improve that, the lifestyle medicine layer of the PAP may be where you stop.

LEVEL 3: AESTHETIC MEDICINE If you want to go further, this is the time to talk about skincare, the first stage of the external elements of the plan. We are all constantly bombarded by adverts and conflicting advice about skincare, so this is the part of the book where I reveal the science behind what they all do, which products are worth spending money on, brilliant brands that don't cost the earth, and which luxuries your skin can certainly live without. Finding the products that work is, for most people, the peak of their PAP journey.

Once you've got great skincare nailed down, you can, if you wish, invest in medical facials that support and boost the great work you're doing on your skin at home.

The next stage is aesthetic treatments that will take your skin to the next level. But how much time and money - *realistically* - are you willing to invest? And what's right for your skin and its needs? There are so many treatments out there, and choosing the wrong one will not only be costly, but will leave you disappointed too. I'll explain which treatments get results and how, as well as which are the best value for money for you, whatever age you are.

Are you thinking of heading straight to the aesthetics chapter? Of course, you can jump in at the top with Botox - or BTX as I will call it throughout, as Botox is merely a brand name - fillers and lasers. Sometimes that kind of kick-start is the push some people need to adopt a more holistic and health-based approach to skin.

But, as I will keep saying, while there is nothing wrong with starting at the top, you will get much better and more long-lasting results by working your way up the PAP, viewing these treatments as the cherry on the top. Once you've got your skin glowing by tweaking your lifestyle, perfecting your skincare and possibly having regular facials, you may even decide that having any more extensive treatment isn't for you.

What beauty means now

Yes, I am a 'Botox doctor', but this is not a hard sell for aesthetics. There is so much you can do to feel beautiful without needles, or even visiting a clinic. That is why the bottom two levels of the PAP are so key. And why, whatever discussions I have with clients and colleagues about cosmetic medicine, we always come back to the very bottom level, Mindset.

I see around 2,000 clients per year, and many of them visit several times each year - so I have really got to know them, to explore their concerns, fears and attitudes to ageing over time. I have walked hand in hand with them, listening hard and genuinely sharing the conflict 'to do or not to do' as the years have passed.

For some, saying NO to 'intervention' reflects a healthy 'pro-ageing' mindset. A good haircut, a well-cut outfit, the right shade of lipstick, a run on the beach, can be all it takes to feel good in yourself.

But I believe that a lot of women are saying 'NO' for the wrong reasons. First, you might be scared. You may have a fear that you'll come out looking like a humanoid, or overdone, or like a reality TV star. I have to say, done well, cosmetic medicine should be invisible. It should just be a tweak, not a transformation. That's why I've called the top level of aesthetic medicine Optimize. I want you to look like the best version of you, refreshed as if you've had a great night's sleep, just come back from a restful trip, exuding confidence, when you leave the clinic.

Second, you might not consider yourself to be 'the kind of woman' who has cosmetic 'work'. Having worked in the industry for 15 years, I can tell you that there is no one type of person who makes up my client base, but this idea goes hand in hand with the concept that these kinds of treatments are a result of the patriarchal view, which suggests that women are only valuable in so far as they are young and beautiful. You might be of the opinion that women shouldn't have to tweak their appearance to feel acceptable in the world.

I agree with the opposite view, in which some people argue that cosmetic injectables and other treatments are no different to wearing make-up - and it's about time the world stopped judging women for having them. Take this view further, and you could even say it's a feminist act to take control of your face, no matter what men, or other women, think of you.

Which view is right? Both, to some extent. I don't believe that women should have to justify their decision to have BTX or any other cosmetic treatments to anyone but themselves. The way I see it, it's your face, your choice and your business.

I hate the idea that women feel they have to do these things to remain relevant. Women's salaries plateau at age 39 while men's continue to rise for another decade. That is truly abhorrent. Women should be judged on the quality of their work, not their looks or youth in the workplace.

But we are living in the world we are living in. And we have been brought up with the beauty values we have. So, within that framework, what will make you feel good about yourself? For most of us, when we feel we look better, we feel better and function better in the world. Whatever you decide to do on the route to that is up to you.

I have struggled for some time to get here; to a place where I feel completely comfortable calling my approach positive ageing. Is my work perpetuating the idea that youth is like currency? Over 30 years ago, Naomi Wolf's *The Beauty Myth* pointed out that as the social power of women has increased, the pressure we feel to adhere to social standards of beauty has increased too. Which has also led me to question whether I am fuelling an industry that sells quick fixes and promises of 'perfection'.

But after many years of reflection, I say not. Not if my clients are coming to this with their eyes wide open, not if they are educated about the facts of treatment, informed about all the costs and options, not if I only recommend treatments that will work for their skin and concerns, not if clients are given the power to create their own treatment plan with me, not if they are told what the actual results can be. I hope this book will do just that without you having to come to the clinic. I want to demystify the ageing process, give you a look behind the curtain at cosmetic medicine, simplify the options you have and the treatments available, so that you are truly in charge.

I do passionately believe in the idea of positive ageing: we really can be happier and feel good about our looks as we get older. I hear so many wonderful stories in my clinic every day about restoring self-confidence with the right skincare and treatments. And that makes me want to tackle the misconceptions and taboos of vanity that surround treatments, the shame or guilt some women have around even considering treatment.

Recently, at the clinic, I've met a new 'breed' of women; a generation of clients who want to look good for *themselves* and do not feel guilty about it. I'm not talking about the very young, trend-led, Insta-face girls. Usually in their 30s, these women take a proactive, savvy approach to ageing and treatment. They want that 'you look really great today' feeling, without appearing artificially younger. They feel no shame about seeking treatments and are not conflicted about their feminism, in the same way as previous generations have been, including my own. I'd argue their attitude can be all of ours.

Positive ageing is not about promoting an impossible ideal. It's not about 'using your assets', or a fear of looking your age. Nor is it about escapism or vanity. It's about self-care, learning to love your face, feeling attractive and powerful in the body you're in, the 'best version of you', brighter, more alive. Wearing make-up because you're allowed to enjoy decorating yourself if you feel like it, but knowing you absolutely don't need to wear it as a mask either. It's about walking into any room not being held back by concerns that you are looking old, tired, sad or angry, not shrinking yourself, owning your space, feeling free.

So, let's harness that *freedom*. Freedom to choose any approach you want, making educated choices whatever you choose. Some of us will accept the grey hair and enjoy it and see it as a sign of our increasing wisdom – others will think that it doesn't suit them and will prefer to dye it. And now the same can apply to our faces, too. Technology and science have developed to give us the freedom to find the appearance that we are truly happy with.

> 'Shave your legs or don't
> Smile from ear to ear or don't
> Liberation has no dress code
> Etiquette or secret dialect . . .
> Take up space
> In any way you choose . . .'
>
> – *Take Up Space*, Vanessa Kisuule

My clients want treatments that no one will notice, and I agree. But I want them to feel empowered by their decision to have those treatments and revel in telling people what they've had. There is no shame in wanting to look after yourself and be your best *you*. And when someone asks you what your secret is? Be proud to mention laser facials in the same sentence as 'good genes' and plenty of sleep. *That* is positive ageing.

How to use this book

I want you to use this book as a working guide, a way to build your own PAP.

That is, as you read through the chapters, take a notebook, or the pages at the back of the book, and jot down the symptoms you might identify with, or parts that speak to you, the changes that seem most possible or are most relevant to your mindset or lifestyle or skin.

You absolutely don't have to do everything – that would be impossible! We don't have the time, energy or money. So we need to prioritize. I recommend you do this by thinking about what you can change this week, what you can change this month, and what you can change this year.

Because every little change can add up to a new habit - and show on your skin.

My wish is, that by giving you the science of the body, skin, skincare and treatments, along with the benefit of my experience and professional opinion, this will empower you to make your own decisions on where to focus your attention. After all, you are the expert on you.

This book is for everyone

This book is written with women in mind, as they make up 5 out of 6 of my clients. But that leaves the 1 in 6 clients who are men, who come to me with broadly the same issues as women, possibly later and possibly in a different order of priority. So you can be confident that the recommendations and treatments in here apply to you, too (with some exceptions in the section on hormones!).

Chapter One

An introduction to skin ageing

There's a difference between the natural process of ageing and what's happening to many of us today.

To be clear: ageing is nothing to be ashamed of, it's going to affect each and every one of us. What I'm concerned with in this book is premature ageing. We're growing old before our time, feeling fatigued and suffering from any number of largely preventable diseases, thanks to a slew of diet, environmental and lifestyle factors that are affecting not just our health, but also our appearance.

Your skin quickly and visibly reflects what is going on, both inside your body and outside, whether that's sky-rocketing stress levels, the growing fog of pollution or skin-damaging UV rays. It's important to know how these issues impact the skin, so you can build on this to understand HOW and WHY you are ageing at a faster rate than you should be. Then later in the book, I'll explain more on the lifestyle changes that reverse this.

Once you know the science, you'll understand how to make the best of your time, money and effort, and not be tempted by products and treatments that turn out to be snake oil. Because when you understand the science of why your face changes, you can learn to slow the process down WITHOUT being tempted and falling for any marketing or misinformation. For example, a £230 serum that promises to treat wrinkles may sound like a miracle but it's almost certainly more hype and hope than sound skin science. When you know over-the-counter products only penetrate as far as the top layer of the skin, you'll know that their ability to address saggy skin or deep wrinkles can be limited. Only prescription skincare will penetrate deep into the dermis, directly addressing collagen damage and depletion. Knowing the structure of your facial skin will help you know which treatments will be effective and so are worth putting into your budget.

The good news is there are plenty of positive changes that will make a difference. And because skin renews itself fast - you grow a whole new set of surface skin cells every 4 to 6 weeks - you'll quickly see the benefits of every one you make.

Appearance is anything but superficial

I meet a lot of clients who struggle with the belief that it's vain or unimportant to worry about appearance. But how you look is, in fact, a crucial indicator of your overall wellbeing. The same processes and imbalances that are giving you wrinkles are also affecting your energy levels, moods and general health.

On a cellular level, skin has a diverse role in so many of the body's systems, from immunity and metabolism to detoxification. So when your body is not working optimally, your skin will suffer - and show it. Healthy body, healthy skin.

Skin is also the chief barrier between the body and the environment, so it bears the brunt of all those environmental stressors from pollution and smoking, to alcohol and UV rays.

Your face can be a fantastic health wake-up call, as it is so often the first place to show signs of strain, much more obvious than clogged arteries or high blood pressure. And because we care about the way we look, it can act as an incentive to make those changes to diet and lifestyle that are making you age prematurely, inside and out.

These are the top 5 issues I hear about when initially meeting clients: 1) Dull and dry complexion. 2) Redness and/or 'sensitivity', sometimes presenting as rosacea. 3) Brown patches, presenting as uneven skin tone, pigmentation or melasma. 4) Wrinkles. 5) Sagging.

All of the above can affect us from our thirties onwards. Each one is the result of a complex interplay between our genes, which includes our gender and ethnicity plus the natural ageing process - the things we can't control - and the things that we can, such as eating a healthy diet or wearing sunscreen. In fact, there's an awful lot we can control - that's what I explain for you first, before looking at skincare and treatments. Achieving great skin starts with changes much simpler than you might think.

Radiant, plump, clear skin comes from inside. There is a limit to what even the best skincare and aesthetic treatments can achieve. If you're knocking back a bottle of wine every other night, smoking and baking your skin to a frazzle, even a top-class aesthetician can't perform miracles.

Indeed, this is why so many aesthetic clinics are branching out into the wellness space, with clients having a parallel programme of skincare and aesthetics with lifestyle health. And that's why this book includes the information I tell my clients about: stress management, improving gut health and nutrition, hormonal balance and environmental defences against UV and pollution, as well as how to choose the right skincare and treatments. If you put in enough time and energy, you'll slow age-induced degradation - and see a big impact on your skin.

Are you inflamm-ageing? How an essential positive, healing response goes awry

The first - and possibly most important - process that's accelerating ageing in your body is inflammation. It's not a new discovery. In fact the Romans described it in the first century: *calor*, *dolor*, *rubor* and *tumor*, also known as heat, pain, redness and swelling. Within seconds of injury, anything from a pulled muscle to a spot, your body mounts this very effective battle cry. Once healing is under way and the body feels safe again, anti-inflammatory chemicals move into the area and mop up.

What is relatively new is the theory that continuous low-level inflammation is the root of so many conditions, from diabetes and depression to cancer, arthritis and Alzheimer's - and the processes of ageing, too.

For the most part inflammation is a healthy part of the healing process, designed to localize whatever is hurting you, and start the process of removing damaged tissue. The problem is that our modern lives result in a mild form of this reaction being triggered multiple times *every* day, whether that's through pollution, UV rays or the internal ravages of the stress hormone cortisol, all of which our body interprets as a series of assaults. From the body's perspective it's constantly under attack, so it switches up our immune response.

Compounding this, our natural anti-inflammatory mechanisms cannot cope. So inflammation never gets switched off. With the immune systems constantly on 'high alert', inflammation becomes a smouldering wildfire . . .

Because we're not taught about inflammation or told about its effects, we assume that changes due to inflammation are a natural part of the ageing process. Aches and pains, gum disease, excess weight, brain fog and tiredness can all be triggered by chronic inflammation, as can many dermatological conditions, including acne, rosacea and eczema, along with premature facial ageing. Think of wrinkles: inflammation damages collagen fibres and interferes with their ability to repair and regenerate.

If you are feeling under par, or if your heart sinks every time you look in the mirror, it is likely not just due to the impact of time, but also to how your diet, lifestyle and environment are ageing you prematurely, inside and out. We will explore this and how to tackle it in more depth in Chapter 3.

Free radical troublemakers

The fuel on the inflammation fire is the damage from substances called free radicals. These are produced by your metabolism - think of them as the body's exhaust fumes - as well as by the impact of UV light and pollution.

When your body is functioning well, most free radicals will be neutralized by antioxidants manufactured by your body, helped along by the extras that come from fruits and vegetables we eat (more information on the best sources in Chapter 3).

But when our antioxidant supply is used up and overwhelmed by an engine that's being constantly revved up by stress, pollution, sleep deprivation, a processed diet, sun, cigarettes, as well as the inflammatory response, the free radicals steal electrons from other cells, destroying them in the process and wreaking havoc.

One favourite target of free radicals is the DNA in our cells. Mitochondria, the power generators in all cells including skin, are also particularly vulnerable. Hit by a high-energy free radical, the cell membrane breaks down and is destroyed. And when the skin's cellular energy producers are hit like this, skin struggles to defend itself, repair and regenerate.

Free radicals love to target proteins and fats too. And that means collagen and elastin, the building blocks of skin, as well as the fats that make up our skin's barrier layer.

The result? Inflamm-ageing. This chronic condition affects every cell, tissue and organ in our body, but on our skin it shows up as all the 5 signs of ageing. That is, dull and dry complexion, redness and/or sensitivity, pigmentation, wrinkles and sagging.

How do we age?

So inflamm-ageing is the trigger and free radicals are the fuel . . . but what is happening in skin?

The following three ageing mechanisms first affect the structure of skin, which in turn affects its function, which finally shows up so you notice it.

Structure -> Function -> Appearance

Defences weaken

As our natural antioxidant supply gradually depletes, accelerated by inflamm-ageing, free radicals run wild and the damage goes unchecked. Added to this, all our skin's support and supply systems, including our blood, lymph and nervous system, which bring essential nutrients and immune cells, start to slow down and become less efficient.

Repairs become faulty

When we're young our bodies can remodel, repair or remove damaged skin cells and other parts, but as we get older this doesn't happen as efficiently. Our elastin fibres, which give the skin its bounce, start to stiffen, so skin no longer springs back as readily as it once did. And there's a gradual decrease of collagen, the supportive protein that gives the skin its structure.

Regeneration powers slow

From our 30s, new collagen and elastin production also slows dramatically. Structural skin cells divide more slowly with each passing decade, slowing by as much as 50% by the time we reach the age of 60. Blood vessels also don't regenerate, which can mean restricted blood flow and our skin cells not getting all the oxygen and nutrients they need.

Under your skin

I'm going to do a quick explanation of your skin's structure first, then relate that to the most common complaints I hear from my clients - including yours, I hope.

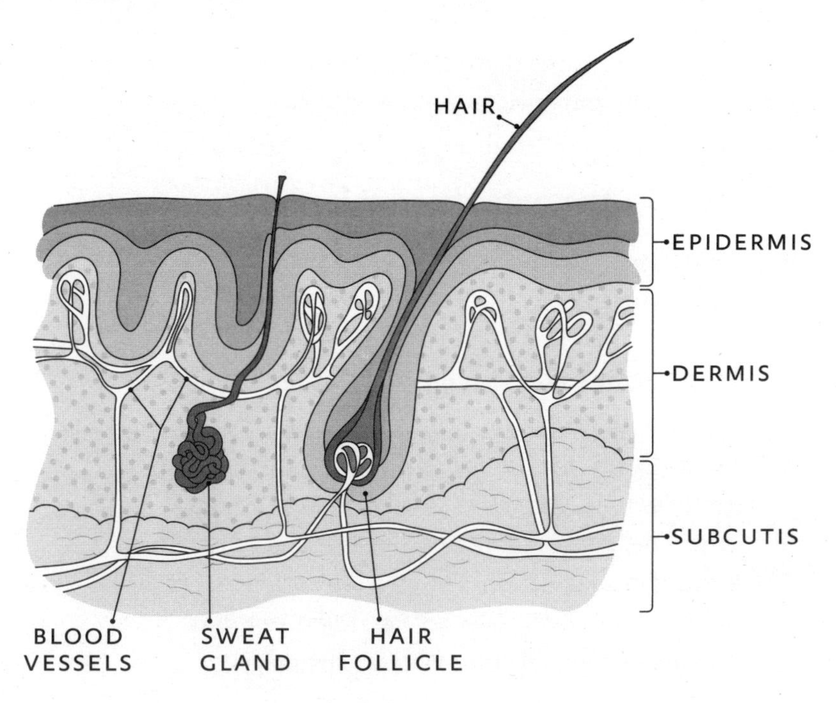

Our skin is a complex combination of proteins, fats, sugars, vitamins, minerals, antioxidants and water. In fact, a whopping 70% of our skin is water. It's a hungry and thirsty organism that needs to protect and feed itself.

Skin has three layers: the deepest is the subcutaneous fat layer or subcutis, then comes the dermis, then the epidermis on top. It also has a microbiome of billions of 'good' bacteria living on the surface.

Whether our skin is radiant and plump or dry, dull and sensitive, or beset with issues like pigmentation, is a combined result of changes at each of the different layers.

At the uppermost level, treating the epidermis will have a dramatic impact on skin clarity and glow. Take a step down to the next level, the dermis, and this is where the skin's youthful bounce is determined, by your stores of collagen, elastin and your skin's inner moisturizer, hyaluronic acid. Pigmentation, wrinkles and early crêpiness and skin sagging can be tackled at both levels, depending on their depth and severity. Underneath the dermis is the deepest layer of skin, the subcutis: fat pads and muscles on top of bone.

1. Epidermis: the outer barrier layer

The job of the epidermis is to keep water in and irritants out. It is made up of:

- **Keratinocytes,** cells that produce keratin, the building blocks of the skin. This is the same tough protein found in hair and nails. Keratinocytes form in the deepest layer of the epidermis, then work their way up to the outermost layer - the stratum corneum. This natural turnover process is called desquamation. The stratum corneum is made up of approximately 15 layers of keratinocyte bricks, surrounded by a mortar of fats and proteins.

- Keratinocytes also produce **natural moisturizing factor (NMF),** a humectant, which means it absorbs water from outside to hydrate skin.
- **Barrier lipids (fats)** are the mortar that surrounds skin's keratinocyte bricks, keeping water in, keeping harmful things out, and helping to give it that plump, supple feel. Keratinocytes are responsible for maintaining these fats - which include ceramides, cholesterol and fatty acids - in a healthy ratio. If either NMF production or your stock of barrier lipids drops, you'll soon notice that your skin feels drier and less smooth.
- **Melanocytes** are the cells that produce melanin, the brown pigment that darkens your skin in response to UV. The melanin acts as a filter, protecting DNA and the collagen that lies deeper in your skin. The melanocytes in darker skin tones produce higher levels of melanin than those in Caucasian skin. The increased concentration of melanin in black epidermis provides a natural SPF of around 13. This protects from some of the harmful effects of UV radiation but not all, so you still need to wear sunscreen. It also makes darkly pigmented skin more vulnerable to irregular pigmentation, especially when the skin is irritated from blemishes or plucking. For more on the differences in ageing between light and dark skins, see the box below.
- The epidermal layer also contains **Langerhans cells**, a type of immune cell. These are the first line of defence against viruses, such as the herpes zoster virus that causes cold sores.

HOW DARKER SKIN AGES

Skins have traditionally been typed according to the Fitzpatrick classification. But that doesn't describe all the differences, only skin colour. Most skincare and skin analysis has traditionally been done on Caucasian/white skins, so we are only now learning that as well as the number of melanocytes, darker skins have a different structure in other ways.

Darker skins tend to have more layers making up their stratum corneum, but lower levels of ceramides and water in the outermost layer of the skin. The dermis tends to be both thicker and more compact, with more and larger fibroblasts. The result is more collagen produced - so fewer wrinkles. The downside to this is a tendency for abnormal scarring, called keloid, where scars can become enlarged and raised, even after a very minor injury. In fact, most clinical signs of ageing, from wrinkles, brown spots and redness to fat atrophy and bone loss, appear a decade later than in lighter skins.

THE SKIN MICROBIOME

The surface of your skin is home to millions of bacteria, fungi and viruses, together called the skin microbiome. These good bugs live in symbiosis with the superficial cell layers of the epidermis, hair follicles, and sweat and sebaceous glands, forming part of the skin's barrier.

There are approximately 1 billion bacteria per square centimetre on our skin, and they are generally not harmful. However, if there's damage to the integrity of the skin barrier, for example from overly harsh cleansing, they may lead to inflammatory disorders such as acne or psoriasis.

The microbiome's composition (the diversity and ratio of different bugs) and function varies by area of the face and by age. For example, in puberty natural shifts in the bacterial mix can trigger the action of sebaceous glands and cause acne. And as you age, the way the balance changes can provoke skin changes in proteins and lipids which accelerate signs of ageing.

A healthy skin microbiome is a key factor in cellular energy generation, so an imbalanced biome is thought to contribute to tired-looking skin, no matter how old you are. It's also important for the functioning of the immune system, essential to protect us from environmental bugs such as skin infections, and to help prevent pro-inflammatory diseases such as eczema.

As a result, probiotic skincare, designed to rebalance the microbiome, is a hot topic. It's an interesting area with big potential, but it's early days and evidence is thin, so I would say it's certainly not a priority you need to focus on. But I am keen to show what we can all do to protect and restore the skin's barrier, including the microbiome - as you'll see in Chapter 4.

2. Dermis: the middle layer

The dermis lies just beneath your epidermis and makes up to 90% of your skin. Its thickness varies from 0.3mm on your eyelids to 4mm on your back. It is where the biggest signs of ageing happen. 60% of the dermis is water. It's also made up of:

- **Collagen and elastin,** the connective tissue of skin. This mesh of thin white collagen fibres and rubbery elastin fibres gives skin its strength, resilience and bounce.
- **GAGs (see page 278),** the water-loving ingredients that surround the collagen-elastin network, hold it together and keep the skin moist and plump. They include one you may have heard of, hyaluronic acid, which can bind up to 1,000 times its volume in water.

- **Fibroblasts**, the key active cells of the dermis, which are responsible for producing collagen and elastin fibres and GAGs.
- A rich network of **blood and lymphatic vessels** that provide essential nutrients to the epidermis.
- As in the epidermis, **melanocytes** produce melanin, our natural sun-protection.
- Sebum is the oil that lubricates both hair and skin. **Oil glands in the dermis** secrete it into **hair follicles**.

3. Subcutis: the thickest, fatty layer of skin

This layer is mostly made from **fat cells.** But these are not passive, they are also an important source of hormones, growth factors, stem cells, immune cells and fibroblasts. It is also made up of:

- **Sweat glands:** This layer is the starting point for our sweat glands, important in filtering out toxins, water and excess salt, and for temperature control.
- **Nerves**, which control our reactions to temperature, touch and pain.
- **Blood and lymphatic vessels**, which deliver nourishment, and act as the clean-up crew for cuts and infections, too.
- **Bones and muscle** are not strictly part of the skin, but they're important as they're the scaffolding of your skin.

How your skin ages

When it comes to looking at the 5 key skin concerns that so many of us worry about, it helps to look at them in the context of the skin's different layers. That way it's easier to understand what's causing the issue, as well as where and how it can best be treated.

For clarity, I've written about these issues as if they stand alone, but of course most people who come into the clinic have more than one issue, each one building on the next.

Problems in the epidermis

As you get older, the epidermal layer, the outermost layer, of your skin thins, so that by the time you're 80, it's half as thick. Melanocytes can fall up to 20% each decade, so the skin tends to become paler and more vulnerable to UV damage and skin cancer. And a drop in Langerhans cells makes you more susceptible to infection, too.

But the epidermis is also where the right skincare and treatments can have a huge impact on skin texture and tone. It's where we start to address these complaints: dull, dry complexion, pigmentation and redness.

Dull and dehydrated complexion

Cause 1: Poor light reflection

Dullness can be due to build-up of dead keratinocytes at the surface of the epidermis as new cell production slows down. This is pretty much a universal problem, post-35 years old. In your 20s, it takes 2 to 3 weeks for a barrier cell to form at the base, work its way to the surface and shed. But by your 40s it can take 4 weeks. The result of this cell build-up is an uneven surface that scatters light, as opposed to a radiant one, where light reflects off a fresh smooth layer of 2-to-3-week-old barrier cells.

THE FIX: Getting a glow back is a quick win for skincare, as the key is exfoliation. I much prefer chemical exfoliators, such as lactic acid, over physical scrubs, which can cause damage and inflammation. They gently dissolve the bonds of the dead skin cells so they fall away to reveal the fresh ones below. These new cells create a surface that both reflects light and absorbs skincare products better. Find out more about which products will suit your skin on page 132.

Cause 2: Leaky skin barrier

As well as dull skin, a leaky barrier can also present as redness and sensitized skin. And when your skin barrier functions less than optimally, it not only allows water to escape, but allows irritants to get in. Although drinking 2 litres of water a day will help your whole-body hydration and detoxification pathways, the hydration of your skin really depends on how well your epidermis holds this water in and stops it escaping. And on how well its cells can top up moisture levels in dry conditions, i.e. good levels of NMF.

Skin barrier function naturally declines over time. Babies don't need moisturizer, because their epidermis has stellar performance and keeps water IN. But after a few decades of a less-than-perfect diet, your barrier layer will begin to underperform as NMF and barrier lipid production dips. For example, lipids - essential fatty acids - come mainly from our diet, which is one reason eating omega-3-rich oily fish is so fantastic for skin. Barrier breakdown is also triggered as a result of trauma, from sun damage, smoke, pollution, make-up and the wrong skincare. So sun-worshippers are definitely at risk, along with anyone who lives in a city. I also see this in skincare junkies who over-exfoliate or use harsh cleansers or astringent toners.

THE FIX: Again, skincare is key here and I will explore what to stop using and what to start using in Chapter 4. But for starters, wear sunscreen, stop smoking, eat more oily fish.

Dry skin

Cause

For most people I see pre-45, skin that feels dry is due to water escaping through a damaged skin barrier, i.e. it's dehydrated, as in the section above. However, for those over 50, dry skin is often due to a drop in sebum production. As you age, sweat and sebaceous glands become less active. Lower sebum levels, a change in composition of the skin's fatty acids, plus sluggish sweat production, especially during menopause, result not only in your skin feeling drier, but in your defences against bacteria being compromised. This can lead to dry, spotty skin. Like a weakened barrier, this can be made worse by harsh cleanser, a common fix which backfires, weakening your skin barrier.

THE FIX: Avoid harsh cleansers, and use skincare with barrier repair ingredients (more of this in Chapter 4). Never sit in direct sunlight, always wear a hat and, again, apply sunscreen.

Pigment change

Cause

Pigmentation and age spots are really just the result of your skin doing its job to protect you. When it perceives a threat, such as UV rays, melanocytes produce melanin, the same pigment that gives you a tan. After 30, as melanocytes decrease and skin colour lightens, you become more susceptible to UV damage and your risk of skin cancer increases. Melanocytes also become ultra-sensitive, with a very low threshold, hence the uneven spots. This is true for all shades of skin.

The hormonal changes which come with pregnancy or with the menopause mean those brown spots could be here to stay. And also, over time, pigmentation issues that start in the epidermis can take hold at a deeper level.

THE FIX: It takes commitment, but quit sunbathing. Also, it's never too late to start using sunscreen and protect your skin from the sun's UV rays (you will hear me say this a lot!). And stop smoking: it provokes pigmentation too. I'll explain more about my multi-pronged approach to pigmentation in Chapters 4 and 6.

Problems in the dermis

The dermis is where wrinkles begin, and that explains why most skincare can't directly treat wrinkles, despite what the adverts tell you, as it doesn't get down that deep in the skin.

However, the right skincare that looks after your barrier function isn't complete nonsense. The healthier your barrier, the better your dermis will function, and wrinkles won't form as easily. Even though skincare doesn't directly affect the dermis, by creating a better-functioning skin in the epidermis it has been shown to impact wrinkle depth, elasticity and collagen levels. I'll discuss more about this in Chapter 4.

Wrinkles

Cause 1: Less collagen and elastin

The number of fibroblasts, the cells of the dermis which synthesize collagen, falls by 10% each decade. By the age of 60 we hardly make any new collagen or elastin. Also, repair mechanisms slow: collagen fibres straighten and become more loosely entwined, while elastin fibres become thinner, longer and slacker, meaning skin has a loss of elasticity with no 'snap back'.

THE FIX: Both collagen and elastin are very vulnerable to blood sugar highs. So please hold off on those sugary snacks as well as high glycaemic foods (see page 90 for details). And skincare helps too: see Chapter 4 for more on this.

Cause 2: GAGs deplete

Every day we use up a third of our stores of hyaluronic acid (HA), which draws in water to keep our skin looking plump. In our youth they are then quickly replenished. But by our 40s we are making about half of what we need. So our HA levels fall, meaning there is less water to keep collagen and elastin moist, meaning they don't have optimal structure or function.

THE FIX: Topical vitamin A (retinoids) stimulates hyaluronic production. The other option is injectable HA skin boosters (see Chapter 7).

CAN HA IN SKINCARE ACT AS A FILLER?

Generally, most HA serums are made up of molecules that are way too big to reach the dermis, so they can't penetrate and add to moisture in the skin. Instead, they sit on the surface. That doesn't mean they are useless; they are a brilliant barrier moisturizer. However, there are now some nano molecule HA serums that claim they can get down to the dermis. Indeed, studies show an impressive improvement in wrinkle depth, skin firmness and elasticity after 8–12 weeks' use. This is a new development, and I'll be watching it closely.

Cause 3: UV rays

Within hours of exposure, UV rays accelerate structural changes to elastin fibres and ramp up the activity of collagen breakdown enzymes (metalloproteinases or MMPs). Collagen breakdown happens across your entire face and body, even in the areas that have not been exposed to the sun. But loss of elastin is generally down to sun exposure, so sunbathing will accelerate this in the areas that you choose to tan. It causes a rubbery, crêpey skin texture and poor spring-back, the kind when you pinch the skin on the back of your hand and it stays as it is.

THE FIX: As always, sunscreen! And limit the amount of exposure your skin gets to direct sunlight.

THE 3 TYPES OF WRINKLES

When you look in the mirror, are wrinkles the first thing you see? Maybe you notice them before anything else, but they don't have nearly the same visual impact on other people. Loss of elasticity, uneven tone and volume loss are far more noticeable.

The basis of the PAP is that you get skin into its best and most glowing condition with the right lifestyle and food, then build on that with the active ingredients in skincare and maintenance treatments. Especially when considering expression lines, skincare can achieve a lot. Even with deeper lines, making sure you get the right building blocks at the bottom of the PAP will mean not only that wrinkles are softened but that people will notice them less, too.

That said, when people think their face doesn't reflect their true self or emotions any more, that is when they want to make a more immediate change. You may be fixating on the fact that you think your deep frown lines make you look grumpy, or nose-to-mouth lines give you a down-in-the-mouth expression or make you look jowly. That's when I will treat the lines using cosmetic treatments. In that case, below are some examples of what I might do cosmetically, although every face is different.

1. Expression lines

This type includes frown lines, forehead lines and crows' feet. The result of repeated muscle contraction, they disappear at rest. They are usually the first lines to appear, from around the age of 30.

THE FIX: A light 'sprinkling' of BTX, to retain natural movement as much as possible. In younger clients, this can also help prevent their appearance. (We will come to a more detailed discussion of BTX in Chapter 8.)

2. **Static lines**
These are due to a decrease in collagen, changes in elastin fibres and decreased GAGs (see page 23). They are visible all the time, not just related to movement. They typically appear on Caucasian skin after 40 and on darker skins 10 years later.

THE FIX: Usually best plumped out with injectable fillers (more on these in Chapter 8). Skin boosters, chemical peels, microneedling and/or laser resurfacing, all of which are explored in depth in Chapters 6 and 7, can also help to soften lines by improving your overall skin quality.

3. **Gravitational lines**
These are the folds that are the result of both fat and bone volume changes and gravity, such as deep nose-to-mouth lines. Depending on your skin type and face shape, they appear from your 30s onwards. High or prominent cheekbones delay this and fat loss will do the opposite.

THE FIX: Again these are best treated with a mix of BTX, fillers and skin boosters, though fillers are the main treatment here. For example, replacing lost volume in the upper part of the face can make nose-to-mouth lines in the lower part less pronounced. (More in Chapter 8.)

Redness from rosacea

Rosacea, a very common chronic inflammatory skin disease, is behind a high number of cases of red and sensitive skin. We don't fully understand it, and it's currently incurable, but it does seem clear that there is a genetic predisposition that makes some people more sensitive to the triggers that result in facial flushing. These can be dietary, alcohol, caffeine and also some parasites found on the skin and in the gut. Eventually, as fragile capillaries become permanently dilated, 'spider vessels' and permanent redness can develop.

THE FIX: Rosacea often responds when you dial down chronic inflammation both on the inside and outside, which can start with simple things like changing your diet and reducing stress. See Chapter 3 for my full rundown of lifestyle changes that could help you, Chapter 4 for skincare advice and Chapter 8 for laser treatment.

Problems in the subcutis

Your overall volume of subcutaneous fat typically diminishes with age, and the way it's distributed also changes. It decreases on the face, hands and feet, and increases in the thighs and abdomen. And while those with black skin are less prone to photo-ageing and wrinkles, even those with darker skin tones are likely to find their cheeks hollow and chins sag as they get older.

Sagging

What clients call 'sagging' can be simply down to dehydration (see page 25), leading to the appearance of crêpiness, especially around the eyes. Or to loss of elasticity, which causes true crêpiness. The common places we see this are 'accordion lines' as you smile, those wide, vertical lip lines. The next stage of sagging shows up as drooping around the mouth, which can progress to jowling.

Regardless of what the scales show, facial fat loss starts in your early 30s. And it plays a far more significant part in bringing people to the clinic than wrinkles. The more fat you have on your face post-40, the younger you look. The early stages of sag include the shrinking of cheek fat pads, the fat pads that sit directly under your eyes and those around your mouth. They can change the instant impression - the 'blink impression' - your face makes, leaving you looking tired or sad. As discussed earlier, the fat on our face is held in the subcutis layer of our skin, which is massively impacted by stress. One important study by UK cosmetic surgeon Rajiv Grover showed that people experienced a 35% drop in facial volume after suffering a traumatic event.

THE FIX: Skincare can help with very early sagging; follow the Reset Programme for Mature Skin (see page 146). But only aesthetic treatments can help tighten the skin at a deeper level. These include radio-frequency, ultrasound or laser treatments. Dermal fillers can be used to compensate for some of the lost volume too (more on these in Chapters 7 and 8).

Sagging from bone and muscle loss

This is when sagging comes from deeper down. As with everywhere in the body, bones and muscles recede with age, from 40 years old in women, slightly later in men. Eye sockets become wider and longer, which can accentuate bags, lines and dark circles. In the mid-face, the nose widens, and marionette lines, shadowing or folds from lip corners to either side of the chin, appear. The angles of the jaw also change, contributing to jowls and neck sag.

Perversely, some facial muscles go through hypertrophy, i.e. they bulk up. This causes deeper frown furrows and, in some people, jaw clenching. This happens in our sleep, but we can also clench our jaws during the day, when we are tense. This can eventually lead to broken teeth and overly developed jaw muscles, which can make your face look more masculine.

THE FIX: A shot of BTX in the masseter (the muscle that runs just in front of your ear, down to your jawline) will help prevent clenching and grinding, as will taking charge of your stress levels (more on this in Chapter 3). Injectable fillers can, to a certain extent, replace lost volume due to bone loss, for example around the eyes and mouth (more on this in Chapter 8).

OTHER SURFACE CHANGES

MILIA: These little white spots appear around the eyes. They are little balls of keratin protein, not pus, so don't squeeze them! Milia can appear at any age, but often become more frequent in middle age. They are also common in newborn babies and in this case will clear naturally.

Regular exfoliation and vitamin A use can help prevent them, but the reason is usually a genetic predisposition. They can be removed manually by trained aestheticians using a needle or radiosurgery.

LARGE PORES: This is often a very subjective diagnosis and another case where what you see in the mirror is often not remotely noticed by your friends or family. If your pores bother you, avoid creams with marketing hype promising instant pore-reduction. Instead look for treatments that reduce excess sebum production and improve elasticity, such as vitamin A (see Chapter 4 for more on this). Or there's 'meso'-BTX, multiple shallow injections of tiny amounts of highly diluted BTX into the dermis, to reduce sebum production and, subsequently, pore size (more on this in Chapter 8).

FACIAL HAIR: In the years leading up to the menopause, the drop in oestrogen leaves testosterone relatively high, which can trigger hair growth. There are many temporary options such as waxing and threading that can work as solutions for some people. But for a long-term fix, laser hair removal is the answer; it's permanent and you don't get all the rashes and irritation that you can get with shaving, threading or waxing. The older lasers couldn't treat all skin types, but the newer lasers can. If you have darker skin, be sure to research an experienced practitioner who is used to treating it.

As the laser works by targeting pigment in the hair, it's less effective for the fine, short, light 'peach fuzz'. This can be tricky to remove, though you could try dermaplaning, which uses a scalpel blade to remove the fine hairs and the dead skin cells. But do remember that some hair on the face is natural: we weren't designed to be hairless.

STRETCH MARKS OR 'STRIAE': A very common occurrence in pregnancy; the hormonal changes make collagen more susceptible to tears as it stretches. Some studies report an 80% chance of developing these in pregnancy.

Sadly, most creams and gels might make your skin feel softer and more supple but aren't proven to work. Although a new method from Secret Saviours has promising research for prevention: you wear a stretchy 'bump band' to support the stomach, off-setting the stresses and strains in the dermis, to prevent the tiny micro tears from forming.

Unfortunately stretch marks are difficult to treat, though microneedling and lasers can be effective, especially if performed early (see page 203 for more information).

TIRED EYES?

This is one of the most common reasons women come into the clinic. As there's usually a combination of factors at play and because it's such a delicate area, it can be complicated to treat. Your tendency towards dark circles and/or eye bags is usually inherited. They're caused by active melanocytes in the dermis giving a blue-grey appearance, but this can also be due to congestion and leaky blood vessel walls. For example, when you have hay fever or a cold, the pressure against blood flow in the area builds up and the under-eyes get darker.

I'll go into the clinic procedures on page 244, but there are some lifestyle changes and skincare ingredients that can help.

- Sleep, although I'm sure you know this. Alcohol and caffeine disrupt the quality of sleep as well as the quantity, and you'll likely know your other triggers too. You might find that the advice on page 63 will help.
- Superficial pigmentation may respond to ingredients such as caffeine, vitamin C and retinol in skincare. Try: Skinbetter Rejuvenate Smoothing Interfuse® Treatment Cream (with caffeine and vitamin C). Medik8 r-Retinoate Eye Serum is a gentle vitamin A, designed for this area (see page 123 for more on vitamin A). Dab a very small amount gently along the orbit bone/upper lid immediately after cleansing.
- Sunscreen is critical in this area - don't ignore it! Even if it's made your eyes water in the past. Skinceuticals Mineral Eye UV Defense is made for the eye area, although you should find a face sunscreen you can wear. Big sunglasses can protect the eye area too.
- If you tend to puffiness, you could try sleeping with an extra pillow, to keep your head elevated. Or apply 2 teaspoons, straight from the fridge.
- Gentle massage will help circulation. Use fingertips to apply pressure on the orbit bone, starting close to the nose and working outwards. Don't pull on or rub skin.

For aesthetic treatments on eyes, see page 244.

CHAPTER ROUND-UP

- Our skin has three layers - epidermis, dermis and subcutis - and by understanding and looking after them we can actively support the health of our skin.
- Most of us are experiencing premature ageing due to diet, environmental and lifestyle factors and hormone imbalance, which can be corrected without intervention.
- Appearance is anything but superficial, and your skin often shows that something is wrong on a deeper level.
- Inflammation is the silent epidemic most of us are living with because of our busy lifestyles.
- The 5 signs of facial ageing are: dull, dehydrated skin, redness, pigmentation, wrinkles and sagging, and each can be explained by changes in the structure and function of the components of these layers.

Chapter Two

Mindset: where it starts

How do you feel about your face?

When people walk into my consultation room, that's the first thing they reveal to me. It's most often negative: they say, 'I look exhausted!' Or they point at a line between their brows and say, 'It makes me look cross', or 'sad', or 'worried'. Or they point at their lower face and say, 'Everything is dropping.'

If any of that sounds familiar, I want to help you change that. My aim is to help you feel good about yourself, all of you. To get away from a negative focus on flaws and towards a positive on how you can look and feel your best, going forward. After all, beauty is a feeling as much as it is physical - how you feel when you look in the mirror and when you walk into a room. What you see in the mirror is so deeply entwined with what's going on in your head. It's not how you look but how you view yourself that impacts your emotions, thoughts, decisions - and quite possibly your quality of life.

If your decision to visit a cosmetic clinic is driven by negativity, it's more likely to turn out to be a disappointment. That's often why you see people who have gone too far: too stretched, too plumped, too frozen. But I hope that by following my *positive* approach to ageing you will be able to find some confidence in your appearance that allows you to feel more in control.

I'd rather people didn't come to clinic because they feel a need to fix something, or to ask for BTX because they feel pressure to conform to what's seen as beautiful or youthful. I want them to come because they want to look after themselves, to feel good about themselves.

That's the purpose of the psychological and self-image questions in this chapter, to set you up for a positive ageing journey. To pinpoint your motivations for reading this book and investing time and energy in yourself, whether you eventually decide if that will involve visiting a clinic, or not.

If you look back to my Positive Ageing Pyramid on page 4, which you will get to know very well as you work your way through this book, you will see how much I value mindset when it comes to positive ageing. It's the basis of everything I do. I hope a positive ageing mindset will inform everything you choose to do from now on, too.

Other people's outsides

We all have physical insecurities. We live in a culture fixated by looks, where we are constantly bombarded with images and encouraged to post photos of ourselves on social media. Of course we are becoming savvier to media manipulations of perfected images, but they still get under our skin.

To compare is human instinct. But now we can compare ourselves to all the most beautiful people in the world, instantly.

We *know* everyone is posting an enhanced version of their 'best life' but somehow we still get sucked in, looking at their bodies, their clothes, their faces, and we feel inadequate. We see their perfected outsides. We don't see their insecurities, their sadness or worries or what they dislike about their looks.

So then throw *ageing* into the mix, both the physical and emotional components of seeing your mortality in the mirror, and that's the point when people feel so insecure that they will often book into a cosmetic clinic like mine.

However, all that emotional baggage is a lot to work on with just needles and creams as tools. All too often, cosmetic clinics are the one-stop-shop for women who are desperate to 'do something'. Along with my medical degree, I have a psychology degree, and I have always felt that listening is one of the most important components of my job as a cosmetic doctor. Just as important as ensuring the best cosmetic results from treatments.

One-to-one at the clinic, I hear so much negative self-talk and deeply felt fear about ageing. Addressing the extremes like body dysmorphia and anxiety that can take a serious toll on your day-to-day life is unfortunately out of the scope of both my practice and this book. But most of us sit on the continuum and know how it can feel. Few of us are immune to the compliment, 'You look so much younger than that.' And most of us are attached to an unrealistic view of our appearance. If you're stressed or unhappy, your appearance can become an all-too-easy focus.

Ageing is a tough call for women. On the one hand we've been fed the line that we are becoming less relevant with each passing year. That our value is in our youth and beauty. And yet on the other, we're also told we must age 'gracefully', that it is shameful and shallow to worry about losing our looks, or to dabble in cosmetic procedures. It's no wonder we're so conflicted.

Is it normal to feel a sense of loss at our passing youth? To worry that we're starting to look a little tired, even after a full night's sleep? Yes, absolutely.

The identity shift brought about by our changing looks is anything but superficial. We no longer have the face we once had, and it can hurt. It can feel like a bereavement of sorts, as one of my clients described it to me. We can be angry, sad and in denial, dealing with all those feelings that come with any loss, big or small, and if you feel like that, it's healthy to acknowledge it.

Of course this probably isn't the whole picture. Think deeply, and you may find a part of you that positively welcomes the shift and the benefits that can come with growing older, whether that is confidence in your proven abilities, the courage that comes from having tackled difficulties, knowledge of the real you and her needs and wants, or being grounded by your tenacity.

By acknowledging the loss we feel, we can start to accept ourselves as we are now, embrace these benefits and move forward into a new phase of life. Rather than looking backward, we can appreciate ourselves as we are, let character and values come to the fore, perhaps not even care quite so much what other people think of us!

So how do we get to this hallowed place of self-acceptance?

First, check in with your internal dialogue. What kind of things are you saying to yourself and about yourself? Are you being kind? Or are you, in fact, being a self bully, shaming yourself with put-downs? Telling yourself, 'You're an ugly old bag.' (I've heard worse in my clinic, believe me.) We wouldn't dream of talking to a friend like this, but somehow these insults trip off the tongue all too easily when we look at ourselves in the mirror.

You don't have to live like this. You can change your thinking habits. This is a bit flippant, but what if I told you that thinking like this is, in fact, ageing you faster? It triggers the stress hormone cortisol, which in turn triggers inflammation!

So please stop beating yourself up. Start by finding something about your appearance you actually like and give yourself a compliment or two. If you can't manage an authentic compliment yet, start by showing yourself a little self-compassion. This is a simple technique of forgiving and understanding yourself, which sounds simple but was shown in a study to have positive results on the self-attitude of acne sufferers.

During the 2-week intervention the participants were encouraged to soften their self-criticism using a number of techniques, for example by writing a compassionate letter to themselves, or writing compassionate statements on prompt cards, such as: 'I feel upset about my acne but it's OK to feel that way', which they read 3 times a day over 2 weeks. After 2 weeks the study participants found their feeling of shame and depression had significantly lessened; not only that, the intervention even reduced the degree to which their acne symptoms bothered them.

Fill in the following sentence on a piece of card or paper, and read it three times a day. Or write it as a note on your phone.

I feel upset about my XXX but it's OK to feel that way.

You might want to turn off the constant stream of perfection that's coming via your phone, too. Because it's not just our internal dialogue, but also the images we look at and how we judge them, that affects how we feel about ourselves. You might find that streamlined online habits can improve your confidence no end. I find Instagram has a unique ability to suck my self-esteem, and I try to spend a few minutes every day weeding out and deleting any accounts that put me in the wrong headspace. I suggest you do the same. Limit the amount of time you spend online and, if you must look at Instagram, seek out body- and age-positive accounts that aim to lift women up, by showing bodies and faces as they really are, with beautiful rolls of flesh, stretch marks, blemishes and wrinkles.

Do you need space to talk?

Experience has taught me that some people really benefit from having support from a therapist when they're struggling with self-image. This is when some deep talking to sort the emotional component of what you are seeing becomes a wiser spend of time and money than any treatments or skincare. Having therapy is part of self-care. It's not about looking backward and digging up the past, but about looking forward to a stronger you.

After doing the quiz on page 45, do worries about your appearance persist? Do these worries stop you socializing or doing things you once enjoyed? If you've tried talking to friends about your feelings and that hasn't helped, or you spend an hour or more a day thinking like this, then it could be time to seek professional help, from a counsellor or a therapist. A good place to start is the Welldoing.org website, which is a brilliant counselling directory of over 1,000 therapists all over the UK. Alternatively, talk to your GP, who may be able to refer you.

How to be anti-ageist

Ageism is still rife in our society. But things are starting to change, largely thanks to the dynamic, powerful and wonderful women who refuse to shuffle off into a dark corner just because they've passed the menopause.

Films, fashion and even some beauty brands are embracing a more inclusive approach. In 2015 LVMH fashion brand Céline celebrated the then 80-year-old author Joan Didion in their ad campaigns, while Rihanna cast stunning 68-year-old model Joani Johnson, alongside several other models of colour, in her 2019 Fenty fashion campaign. Dove has long since celebrated women of all ages, shapes and sizes, and MAC flies under the banner of 'All Ages, All Races, All Genders' as the world's most-followed make-up brand.

But in the UK, only 5% of TV presenters are women over 50, and in films, female leads are still on average 4½ years younger than their male counterparts. However, things are improving here too. When promoting *The Crown*, in which she played a deliciously provocative Princess Margaret, Helena Bonham Carter extolled the virtues of growing older. 'When I turned 50, I worried it was downhill all the way,' she said, speaking to *Harper's Bazaar*. 'But it's been quite the opposite. I don't think I've ever been happier or more fulfilled. This huge blooming of television means character-driven stories, so there's a lot of choice and a lot of work. When I was young, you were considered "older" over 30.'

Other cultures do ageing better than we do in the UK. Take the French. Rather than trying to turn back the clock, their approach is to look good at whatever age they are. 'In France, there is a saying, "Life begins at 50", whereas in the US I have heard women in their 30s complain they are too old,' Mireille Guiliano, author of *French Women Don't Get Facelifts*, has said. Women in their 40s and 50s are still considered desirable in France, and French men happily flirt with them, says Guiliano. Though I'd argue the beauty ideal includes the 60s and beyond - as it should. Look at Catherine Deneuve (age 76), Jane Birkin (73), Isabelle Adjani (65) and Juliette Binoche (56).

But look deeper, and you'll discover that the French take skincare seriously from an early age. A survey by the market research company Mintel found that 33% of French girls between 15 and 19 are already using anti-ageing or anti-wrinkle creams. And they are certainly dabbling in medical aesthetics, according to my French colleagues. It's just that the trend there, as in my clinic, is for 'natural' or 'Baby Botox', as it's often known, and skilfully placed fillers, which are so subtle as to be unnoticeable. The goal is to look as natural as possible, rather than to have an ever-smoother complexion.

You may or may not want to have this kind of invasive treatment. That's not the point. But there are three things I think we could adopt from the French model. First, it's not vain or silly or shallow to care about the way you look. It's a form of self-care. Second, you're allowed to take it seriously, in terms of commitment, time and money. And last, you can look and feel good at any age.

The mindset quiz

Getting real about your motivations, expectations, and commitment are the keys to a healthy mindset around your looks. What do you see? Why do you want to change it? How far will you go?

This is a version of an exercise all our new clients complete, a series of questions to ask yourself, to reflect on, to check in on yourself. Doing the quiz is designed to prompt you to consider how you might address any feelings or thoughts that come up.

Sit and look in the mirror. What do you see? Draw or write on the picture below or list overleaf.

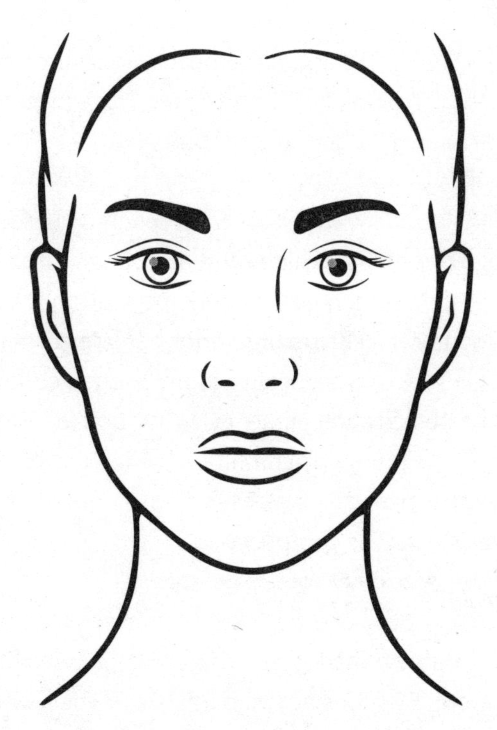

Put it in words. Put it on paper. Sit with it.

1.
2.
3.
4.
5.

How do you feel about it on a scale of 1–5 (1 being happy and 5 being unhappy) and why?

1.
2.
3.
4.
5.

What are your best features? What do you like about your appearance?

1.
2.
3.
4.
5.

If you could change one thing, what would it be?

Do you think this would make you feel more confident?

Would you be more socially active?

Would you wear less make-up?

Would you leave the house without make-up?

Would you apply for a new job?

What do friends and family say they find beautiful about you? What do people compliment you on?

What 5 things would you do differently if you looked the way you want to (while still being you!)?

1.
2.
3.
4.
5.

What would happen if you did each one of those things now?

1.
2.
3.
4.
5.

Positive mindset tweaks

If you're seeking 'intervention', a lifestyle shake-up, upgrading your skincare or exploring medical aesthetics for any of the following reasons, it's a sign there's an emotional component you need to unpick. Here are some of the common emotional triggers that I see in my clients and my advice for how to deal with them.

1. I feel as though I'm stuck in 'the Waiting Room', where my dreams for a better life hinge on improving my appearance.

WHAT TO DO: Really, it's not your appearance that is holding you back, but how you feel about it. This is where you need to deal with the real underlying issues first, which is likely to come down to self-esteem and mindset. Do the quiz, above.

This is my favourite inspirational quote: 'Whatever you do, or dream you can do, begin it. Boldness has genius, power and magic in it.'

Those 5 things that you would do differently (see your scribbles above) - put how you feel about your face and body aside for a moment, and now write down one thing you can do right away, to show how you can take your first step towards making them happen.

This Book Will Make You Feel Beautiful, by Dr Jessamy Hibberd (psychologist) and Jo Usmar, is an excellent practical guide to help improve body image and combat self-doubt in order to feel more confident in your own skin.

The book details many strategies/techniques/exercises (based on CBT) for helping improve body image, etc. One of them is about tackling 'thought crimes'. One exercise asks you to notice when you ignore, dismiss or explain away compliments. This is so interesting to do, next time someone compliments you. Do you bat it away, automatically? Make a joke of it? Say it's not true? Instead, could you practise trying to accept compliments? Or at least not to contradict the person who's complimenting you? Now you've started doing this, you'll notice so many other people doing it too.

2. I feel vain and/or guilty for spending time and money on myself - it's such a waste.

You not wasting anything. You are spending time on you. And this is a vital part of building self-esteem.

WHAT TO DO: Try to get out of autopilot and become more aware of where the judgement and/or guilt is coming from. One technique that I've learned from Dr Tara Swart - whose book *The Source* is truly life-changing - shows how we can all harness the potential to transform our minds and attract and seize the opportunities that pass us by every day.

Focus on the issue that's bothering you. You could visualize spending time and money on yourself, perhaps going to an aesthetic clinic, going for a haircut or colour, or a pedicure or massage, depending on where you are stuck.

- What thoughts come into your head? That is your rational or logical mind speaking.
- What is in your heart? (I often place my hand on my heart.) That is the emotional you speaking.
- Finally, put your hand on your stomach. What does your gut tell you? That is your intuition speaking.

There are so many layers of imprinted thoughts and feelings about what we should feel and think that come from childhood, our families, the culture we grow up in, our peer group. But this technique short-circuits them for me, so I realize what *I* want. And it's amazing what comes up when I do this exercise.

3. Instagram is really getting me down. Everyone looks so young and beautiful, successful and confident.

WHAT DO TO: Switch off! Or, as I've said, edit your feed. Or you can decide to look at it less, perhaps only once a day with time limits, or even once a week. Honing your account so it shows you only the people who make you feel good will make you feel a lot better.

4. Help, I need a miracle fix. I've got a big event next month and my ex is going to be there.

WHAT TO DO: This isn't what you want to hear, but real improvements take time. Yes, you can have a BTX, filler or laser treatment now, but it's not the answer. From diets to winning the lottery, we are sold quick fixes almost every day of our lives. But the reality is, there are none. To get the best results, you will need to take time and make investments.

Lifestyle changes do not carry the costs or risks associated with aesthetic medicine, but behavioural change is hard. The rewards will be life-changing, so this is always where I encourage you to start. We will explore how lifestyle can affect your skin and ageing in detail in the next chapter.

Lifestyle medicine is not just preventative, but can actively reduce the impact of inflammation and other ageing factors. If you are looking to go further, say to turn back time on some of the Factor 2 oil-provoked damage from your teenage sunbathing years, when you've got the basics of skincare and lifestyle down, you might want to look into aesthetic medicine.

If you decide to do that, seek in-depth, personalized advice to nail down your expectations to results that are realistic and commit to an annual plan that suits your budget. There is absolutely no point in creating a wishlist of products and treatments that you cannot afford financially or time-wise. Apart from anything else, the stress of this is totally counter-productive for your skin!

Be realistic with whichever avenue you go down and you will see results. I promise.

5. I've seen Dr X,Y and Z but it hasn't worked, i.e. I don't feel better.

WHAT TO DO: There is a small possibility this may indicate body dysmorphia. BDD (Body Dysmorphic Disorder) is a body image anxiety disorder, where sufferers focus on a perceived flaw in their appearance, becoming convinced that they are ugly or deformed. It affects 1–2% of the population, but I think it is hugely under-diagnosed, as it's so often considered a physical issue, not a psychological one. If this sounds like you, you may want to consider therapy (see page 43).

What's more likely is that being unsatisfied after treatment means you've gone straight to the top of the pyramid, rather than building the foundations of healthy skin: cutting stress, getting the right skincare, eating well and looking after yourself.

Clients are always asking: 'When should I start having X, Y, Z aesthetic treatment?' I answer their questions on the treatment in detail and send them away with a detailed pro and con analysis and having weighed up the benefits and risks. I tell them that one morning, they will wake up and have made their decision. Sometimes this is not to have the treatment at all.

I cannot stress enough how important building a healthy mindset and lifestyle are before moving up the pyramid to this stage. Without this, you can have the absolute best facials and injectables, but they won't make a difference to the way you feel about your looks. That's what the next two chapters are about: building the foundations of positive ageing.

CHAPTER ROUND-UP

- Beauty is a feeling as much as it is physical – what you see in the mirror is deeply entwined with what's going on in your head.

- We all deal with ageing in different ways.

- Watch your internal dialogue. Is it overwhelmingly self-critical and negative? What can you do to change that? Look at 'detoxing' your Instagram feed.

- Deal with - or at least be aware of - any underlying mental or emotional issues before considering any intervention, even a skincare upgrade, diet and lifestyle changes or at-home treatments.

- Exploring motivations, expectations and commitment are the key to a good aesthetic outcome. It's OK to say yes. It's OK to say no. Make it an informed decision.

Chapter Three

Lifestyle medicine

There are 3 questions I now ask every new client: Do you wear sunscreen? What's your sleep like? What are your bowel habits? And I want to know *all* the details. You'd likely expect the first two questions in a skin clinic. But the last one? Not so much.

Why do I want to ask these questions? From the earliest days of practising as an aesthetic doctor, there was one phrase I kept hearing: 'It's all happened so suddenly.' Clients would complain that their looks deteriorated significantly over 1 to 2 years.

When I asked them to tell me more, I discovered it was often after a period of intense stress. Sometimes this was mainly mental, such as divorce, bereavement, professional upheaval, lockdown, sometimes physical, such as pregnancy, sleepless breastfeeding nights, the menopause, illness. And specifically during lockdown, clients reported this change after just 6 months.

It got me thinking: how much is stress contributing to visual ageing? And what, if anything, can be done to somehow compensate and take care of our skin before, during and after tough times?

The mind-stress-beauty connection

As a doctor, I knew skin was a key organ of elimination. I knew it was therefore linked to every other system in the body. As I started to look into it, I discovered research showing how stress of all kinds has a knock-on effect in every part of our body and mind. It can stop us eating well, but it can also stop us absorbing nutrients. It can disrupt our sleep and prevent us from finding the time or energy to exercise. And it directly affects our hormones, and even the expression of our genes. All of these things show up on our skin.

This was my introduction to lifestyle medicine, and how it affects our skin, which is the basis of this level of the PAP. Of course, as a cosmetic doctor I am interested in more conventional advice too: why you need to wear sunscreen because the evidence for sun damage is inarguable, and why smoking is the enemy of skin. At the same time, in this chapter, I want you to go deeper and look at your lifestyle from a more holistic angle.

I have divided suggestions into four parts for ease: Stress, Nutrition, Hormones and Environment, although they all affect each other. This level of the PAP is about you discovering the root causes of any skin issues, giving your skin the best healthy foundation possible. While the advice I give will have an overall impact on your health, it is targeted in a way that will show up on your skin. The results won't be instant, but they will be profound.

In a society filled with fad trends and quick fixes, we need to take more of a long-term view. This chapter is not about the inevitable impact of time and genetics, but about showing you how diet, lifestyle, hormones and environment are ageing us prematurely, inside and out. Sugar, stress, a sedentary lifestyle, all trigger inflammation and hormonal imbalances, and the more out of balance you are, the faster you will age. The wonderful news is that simple tweaks here can make a huge difference, supporting your body as it transitions through age.

We spoke about inflammation in Chapter 1, and how so many of us in the Western world are living with this chronic condition that is not only making us feel sub-par, but accelerating the ageing process, inside and out. You know instinctively that your appearance reflects your overall health. And when you don't like what you see in the mirror, it adds to your stress and so to not feeling good. In this chapter, the 4 parts are each about building anti-inflammatory healthy habits that bring the added benefit of giving you healthy-looking, glowing skin.

This chapter is also about redressing the popular myths I am asked about all the time, such as: Is running bad for your face? Is chocolate making your acne worse? And do supplements actually make any difference?

As you read this chapter, the changes I'm advocating may sound like a lot. But you can do as many as you wish, or just a few. Some of the suggestions are targeted for different skin concerns, so that may help you decide. But whatever tweaks you choose to make, they'll make a difference, not only to your skin but to your overall wellbeing and, I hope, happiness.

1. Stress

I've put the stress section first because it's the very foundation of internal skincare. If you can set up some support structures that allow you to get good sleep and regular relaxation, you are setting yourself up to feel good, to have good skin and to have the headspace to make other healthy changes, too.

The stress response, like inflammation, is a protective mechanism that goes awry in our modern lives. It is beautifully designed to protect you from a hungry lion, but unfortunately that lion is in our heads these days; a relentless battle against all the stress of our day-to-day. Modern stress is cumulative, chronic, and exhausting.

My clients live over-scheduled, over-committed lives - and it's likely you probably do, too. That's not a criticism, but I'd love you to think of yourself more, to decide to practise all the techniques that are proven to support your body during stress. Because stress definitely affects appearance. And when you're not happy with your appearance, you're not happy in general. It can be a vicious circle.

I define stress as when demands placed on you exceed your perceived ability to cope. When this happens, your thoughts, feelings, behaviours lead to physical changes that aren't good for skin. Hence all those people who come to me during and after a big stress.

It's also important to note that stress is not just emotional, it can be physical or chemical. If you have a gut or viral infection, or if you over-exercise - this is a stress on the body. And stress doesn't just show as feelings of anxiety, hopelessness or pressure, its presentation is biological too. That's why it will present as altered bowel habits, headaches, chest tightness, brain fog, for example. Think back: how many times have you experienced a physical stress symptom over the last month?

More stress -> more inflammation -> chronic stress accelerates ageing

The science: when stress goes wrong

Just like the healing inflammatory response that becomes damaging when it keeps happening, stress is great when it comes in short bursts. But it's when it becomes chronic that it goes haywire, and our bodies see the effects.

So how does it work? When your brain perceives an attack - which could be on your body but is likely something more abstract, such as a difficult work situation or a clash with a family member, your brain signals to your adrenals, the tiny glands that sit on your kidneys, to produce adrenaline. Your heart rate goes up and your big power muscles are flooded with blood, ready for fight or flight. Blood is diverted into your body and away from your skin. This is where the phrase 'white with fear' comes from. Your heart starts racing and you're ready to take action against whatever is threatening you. Again, very useful if there is an animal chasing you or a sudden deadline you need to meet at work. But this stress reaction isn't sustainable over a long period of time.

WHEN SHORT STRESS BECOMES LONG STRESS

The body should get a clear signal when the battle is won or you've escaped the predator. But, this doesn't happen in our always-on modern life. Just as with inflamm-ageing, when stress never drops, cells become resistant to the messengers and won't switch off.

If the 'threat' continues, a SWAT team of stress hormones kicks in, cortisol being the chief one. The main stress-response system mobilizes its troops to prepare for battle, such as rallying immune cells to fight invaders. The body builds energy reserves by breaking down tissues and blocking or slowing processes that are not critical for the fight for survival, such as new cell synthesis and repair. That includes the repair of skin and its barrier and the production of new skin cells.

What is the physical result of this? Blood pressure stays up, permanently. The body tends to store fat, in particular visceral fat, the fat around your organs. This is when TOFI (thin outside, fat inside) can happen: you may not put on weight but your waist expands. Your immune system takes a hit and you become more susceptible to bugs. And vital repair and regeneration resources aren't directed towards skin.

Why is our appearance so affected by stress?

Skin is not just a passive barrier to all that's going on inside us. It plays a super-active role in the body's stress response. It is directly involved in the response from the very beginning; perceiving the warning sign of danger, for example a change in temperature or pain. Skin cells also produce their own stress hormones independently of the rest of the body, so every time you are under stress, your skin is directly responding. And then it is affected by the body directing its focus away from the skin barrier.

The very nature of how skin is built, constantly in a cycle of breakdown-repair-reproduction of all its components, means it's always being rebuilt. It's normally very effective at this process. That is, except when the physiological pressures of stress play havoc with skin repair mechanisms. In fact, having high levels of cortisol, a natural steroid, actually leads to the same effects on skin as long-term use of medical steroid cream: thin, shiny, lifeless skin.

How does stress show up on your face?

You won't be surprised to hear that stress is a contributor to all 5 of the key signs of ageing, as well as acne.

Dull, dry complexion

Reduced lipid production and cell turnover leads to a weaker skin barrier as well as a build-up of dead cells on the skin surface. This, in turn, leads to more water being lost and skin becoming dehydrated. As long-term stress raises cortisol, it lowers your production of oestrogen, a sort of mini menopause, if you like. And this not only lowers the production of new collagen and hyaluronic acid in the dermis but reduces the activity of sebaceous glands and, subsequently, production of sebum at the surface, leaving skin looking dry.

Redness

Stress leads to your blood vessels becoming more fragile, and therefore more likely to dilate and burst. Stress hormones also trigger the release of histamine by skin mast cells; this causes inflammation, which you'll notice as red, hot and itchy skin. Mast cells are also a key producer of hormones that stimulate even more stress hormone, so that's a double whammy.

If you have any existing tendency to an inflammatory skin condition - such as eczema, rosacea or acne - stress can tip the balance, either provoking it or making it worse. And stress in this case can be external, such as pollutants, UV, heat or cold, but also internal.

Pigmentation

Stress stimulates the production of many inflammatory chemicals, including IL-1 alpha, which stimulates the production of the melanin-stimulating hormone (MSH). MSH triggers an enzyme, tyrosinase, to produce more melanin (brown pigment). But tyrosinase powers formation of more cortisol as well as melanin. Also, because stress reduces natural cell turnover, melanin-filled cells will linger at your skin surface for longer.

Wrinkles

Not only does the sustained high level of cortisol from long-term stress stop the production of new collagen, but it also breaks it down and makes it harder to repair. It affects elastin formation and repair, too. The result is thin, weak skin - and, over time, the formation and deepening of wrinkles.

Sagging

This is initially due to a drop in hydration, then in collagen and elastin levels. But stress can also trigger fat loss and bone loss. These layers are the scaffolding of the face. Raised cortisol levels over time interfere with new bone cell formation, so that more bone tissue is broken down than is deposited.

Acne

Adult acne often has its roots in underlying stress, in particular in the raised CRH (cortisol releasing hormone) and compromised gut health that comes with stress (more on this in the next section). Oil glands go into overdrive, and using overly aggressive or drying skincare and picking or squeezing only makes this problem worse. All of the above drive inflammation, and because your skin talks to your brain, this leads to even higher increased stress levels in the entire body (systemically). And so the cycle continues.

CASE STUDY

Helen, aged 44, came to me because she wanted treatment for large, cystic spots and a sore, red face. She told me she was never spot-free. I diagnosed her with acne rosacea, which is an inflammatory condition of the oil glands and hair follicles. In the early stages your cheeks flush more readily, in the middle stages you develop dilated veins in your cheeks, then later on skin can become inflamed and pustular.

Helen wanted me to prescribe Roaccutane and anything else that would give her a quick fix.

She was disappointed when I told her that the first step would be a stress and diet overhaul. I have seen, again and again, that inflammatory conditions like rosacea can't just be treated from the outside.

As a professional and single mother, Helen was the epitome of a woman burning the candle at both ends. I told her that she needed to give more time to herself, to work on her stress levels. She wanted antibiotics, but it was clear from her symptoms that her gut wasn't functioning well, so I explained that it would be a good idea to try other routes first.

Lockdown gave her an opportunity to change, and she seized it. Helen told me that, in fact, working from home gave her time to pause and rethink her life, to get her client list down to a manageable number. She began to exercise outdoors and do online classes at home, rather than force herself to go to the gym every day, which she realized she'd never really liked. She wasn't pushing herself nearly as hard as she had been.

Helen was already tracking her sleep with an Oura ring, wearable tech that also monitors stress. Once she no longer had to travel to see clients, or to stay in hotels, she noticed she felt less stressed. She made sure she stopped work every evening at 7 p.m. She took the time to monitor her sleep and make sure she had regular bedtimes, and noticed she was sleeping better too. Not having to commute, she found she had time to cook from scratch and eat better as a result. She had a blood test that showed she was deficient in vitamin D, so she started taking supplements. I also advised her to take omega-3 supplements, for their anti-inflammatory effect.

With Helen's skincare, I took her back to a few key basics, and told her she wasn't allowed to use the multiple harsh products she'd panic-bought. I put her on the Intervention programme for acne (see page 154 for the full programme), which includes salicylic acid to exfoliate the skin, sunscreen to protect the skin, and prescription tretinoin (vitamin A) to renew skin.

After 4 months of her new lifestyle, Helen's skin looked so much better, she didn't need antibiotics or Roaccutane. When she first came to me, she wasn't able to have laser treatments for the dilated vessels that come with rosacea (see more on laser in Chapter 8), as it's best to perform them on skin that's not inflamed or pustular. But she has now started a course to reduce the residual redness from years of inflammation (see page 242 for more on this treatment). Helen thinks that at some point her work schedule will have to become much busier again, but now she has seen the positive impact from sustained changes to her habits, eating, exercise and skincare, she's motivated to keep them up.

The skin calm plan

You've probably read plenty of advice about how to combat stress. Perhaps you've tried some different approaches. If you already have your techniques for doing this, if you know which habits work for you, keep doing it. Whether it's a morning walk, a meditation app, yoga, cooking or colouring, crack on!

Below, I've put down what I've seen works for the clients I see in clinic - and I include what works for me, too. As you'll see, these may seem like the most basic of changes, but I've seen them make a profound difference to clients' skin. The essential elements I recommend are: stress reduction through breathing, sleep and movement. The next layer is: time in nature, gratitude, friendships, taking time for you. You don't have to do everything - but do something.

What you need may already be obvious to you. If you are busy with a baby, you probably need more sleep. If you are glued to your desk all day, you need to commit to moving more.

It's worth it: managing stress has been shown to decrease inflammation in the body and increase cellular repair, as well as improve gut health, digestion and nutrient absorption (more about this later in the chapter), as well as raising your defences to environmental stressors and re-balancing your hormones. Remember, all of these things are interconnected, and all of them affect your skin. For example, boosting levels of B-endorphins, one of your body's 'happy hormones', slows down the natural decline in the production of keratin, the key protein of your epidermis.

Breathe better

This is not meditation, or even mindfulness. And it is not difficult, I promise. Breathing is the first thing I ask clients to focus on, because it is, bar none, the simplest way to reduce stress levels. There are multiple benefits for skin if you learn to breathe better. Deep breathing flips the switch from fight or flight mode, which is ruled by the sympathetic nervous system, into relax mode, ruled by the parasympathetic nervous system, in less than a minute.

As you breathe, you bring oxygen into your lungs, and expel carbon dioxide. Oxygen is vital for converting food to energy. It's used for the production of ATP (adenosine triphosphate), the fuel that transports cellular energy from every cell's generators, the mitochondria. Plus the lymphatic system requires breath and movement to pump. It collects cellular waste, delivers nutrients, and helps destroy pathogens that are no good for the skin.

1. Close your eyes. And breathe. Try breathing out as if through a straw. You may only have time for 3 breaths. Ideally at least 10. No app required. No need to lie down. No need to time, chant, force your mind to clear. Your attention will automatically be drawn to just how tense you didn't realize you were. Just breathe. Repeat as often as you can.
2. A handy tip, one that works for me, is to leave small coloured stickers by light switches, on the taps, on door handles, that remind me to stop and breathe.

3. Try this 2 x breathing technique. Breathe in for 2 counts, breathe out for 4, then breathe in for 3 counts, then out for 6.
4. Mind shift. This is harder, but simply try to stop focusing on whatever is consuming you and bring your attention to your breath, as it goes in and out. This may help you to pull back and find some more perspective, so you feel more at ease.
5. If you are interested in taking this another step on, and trying meditation, the Insight Timer app is free, and with 60,000 meditations from some of the best teachers in the world, you'll definitely be able to find one or more you love.

Sleep better

You know if you need to sleep more, and more deeply. You're the one who falls asleep when you sit in front of the TV, who struggles to keep her eyes awake at her desk. Maybe you keep going by mainlining coffee in the morning or tea and chocolate in the afternoon, or even wine in the evening.

I ask all my clients about the length and quality of their sleep because it's so vital, affecting every system of the body and mind. Sleep should be your time for cellular repair and hormonal maintenance. Having enough sleep will lift your mood and give you stamina. Not having enough will show on your skin, fast. But so will any improvements you can make to your sleep patterns.

Your sleep-wake cycle, also known as your circadian rhythm, has a huge impact on the regulation of key hormones, including thyroid and growth hormones as well as sex hormones. Keeping to a regular rhythm of bedtime and waking up, ideally in tune with the 24-hour solar day, is good for hormones and therefore for beauty too (see more about skin and hormones in the hormone section, page 96).

Deep sleep, the most restorative and rejuvenating sleep stage, is essential for growth and repair, new collagen production and the repair of some of the DNA damage from UV exposure during the day. You do repair during the day too, but the growth hormone spurt you get during deep sleep gives a big boost. The amount of deep sleep you get is personal and can vary from none, to a third of your total sleep time. On average, it's 15-20% or 1-1½ hours a night. Deep sleep significantly declines as we age.

A 2018 study by the US military showed that sleep helps wound healing, which you could think of as an extreme form of the damage our skin encounters every day. The sleepers' wounds healed faster than those of the sleep-deprived, even when the non-sleepers were given supplements that effectively lowered the inflammatory mediators known to slow down wound healing.

Sleep deprivation disconnects your brain from your stomach, leading to food cravings and mindless eating of foods that don't help skin, such as sugary or salty snacks. One reason is that levels of two appetite hormones, ghrelin and leptin, get out of balance when you're sleep-deprived. Many studies show that sleep deprivation results in a rise in the hunger hormone ghrelin and a drop in the fullness hormone leptin. So you feel hungrier.

At the same time, less deep sleep means low growth hormone. And growth hormones tell cells to use fat over carbohydrates for energy. The end result, over time? Higher fat, lower lean muscle. And so begins the vicious circle I see in clinic all the time: poor sleep -> poor mood-> overeating, over caffeinating -> ditching exercise plans -> poor self-image.

My deeper sleep plan

- I need at least 7 hours sleep per night. The amount we each need is individual, but most of us need 7-9 hours. Work backwards to find your bedtime. I like to wake before the family at 6 a.m., so I need to be asleep by 10. Remember, none of us sleep with 100% efficiency.

- A bedtime ritual. I use my skincare to signal to my body that it's bedtime. This is when the power of massage, oils and lovely scents really has a benefit.
- Bedroom prep. Make sure it's dark, quiet, cool, with no piles of washing, shopping or work. Also, ideally no working, shopping or scrolling in the bedroom for at least an hour pre-bed, if you can help it, a personal electric sundown. The light from devices, in particular the blue light portion, is thought to decrease levels of the body's natural sleep hormone, melatonin. Melatonin is a hormone secreted by your pineal gland which preps you for sleep by lowering your blood pressure and core temperature in preparation.
- If I drink coffee, I won't have one after midday. Some people can handle afternoon caffeine, but others - in particular those who have a gene called CYP1A2, which slows down caffeine metabolism - really cannot! You'll very likely know if caffeine affects your sleep.
- I try to have eaten by 8 p.m., as it's best to have no food for 2-3 hours pre-bedtime. Food makes the body produce insulin, which signals to your body to stay awake.
- Thirty minutes before I get into bed, I start to wind down with a cup of comforting caffeine-free tea, some reading, a bath. And definitely no work, as I know that sends my mind into overdrive. Cortisol levels are meant to be highest in the morning, then lowest at around 11 p.m. It's the fall in cortisol that triggers a rise in sleepy melatonin, so at this point you want to do all you can to keep cortisol levels low - so no late-night alcohol or anxiety, ideally.
- On those glorious days when I have a chance to nap, I do it after lunch, as this is when temperature and cortisol drop, roughly 8 hours after waking. If you often reach for tea and a biscuit to keep you going at this point, you are tired and having a 20-30 minute nap would be better. If you are not an insomniac, this shouldn't affect your regular sleep

pattern. But I will always try not to have a nap in the evening, or a lie-in, as these throw out your circadian rhythm, so you are more likely to have trouble getting to sleep.

Exercise smarter

Find a form of exercise that you enjoy doing. And, if you can, do it 3 times per week for 30 minutes. But even a brisk walk for 30 minutes every day is great.

Do not increase your stress doing something you hate. Do not increase your stress doing something too strenuous. This is especially true if you are already sleep-deprived because of hormones, the menopause, children or work. If that's you, do not push your body hard. HIIT (high intensity interval training) and hardcore running will only further raise cortisol levels.

Try not to save workouts for the weekend. The stress release from exercise lasts 24 hours, and you need it during the week too!

Why am I so keen on it? Exercise is such a powerful full-body anti-ager, including your skin. Studies repeatedly show that exercise reverses ageing at a cellular level, helping genes work as they did when you were younger. One fascinating study of 65 year+ volunteers exercising over a 6-month period showed not only a 50% increase in strength in their thigh muscles, but also many positive genetic changes.

Exercise calms you. The stress response primes us to leap into action - but 95% of the time there's no lion to fight or even any running away needed. That's why exercise is so cathartic: it releases all that revved-up energy inside you.

It also gives you a natural high by increasing levels of feel-good endorphins. These not only boost mood, but have anti-inflammatory benefits, directly lowering cortisol levels, and acting as a natural pain reliever. Exercise also induces the body's production of natural cannabinoids, which are thought to have a relaxing and balancing effect on mind and body, hence the popularity of CBD oil.

THE AGE REVERSAL BENEFITS OF EXERCISE

1. Changes the way over 200 genes work, reversing age-related deterioration in function across all systems of the body, including immunity and brain as well as increasing body strength, muscle mass and bone density.
2. Gives you a healthy glow by boosting circulation and lung capacity - which means a better delivery of nutrients and oxygen to cells and skin.
3. Sweating helps detoxify the body. Many industrial toxins, including heavy metals, pesticides, petrochemicals, are excreted through sweat.
4. There are structural skin benefits too - one study shows how exercising for 30 minutes, twice a week, can result in a thinner stratum corneum (which means better glow) and a thicker dermis (which means fewer wrinkles).
5. Lowers blood sugar levels, leading to less skin caramelization (see glycation/'sugar sag', page 89).
6. Boosts growth hormone and so improves cellular repair and regeneration mechanisms.
7. Promotes bone growth, combatting the facial bone recession (and sagging) that happens with age.
8. Lowers inflammation, so reduces the effects of inflamm-ageing generally.
9. Boosts gut health by encouraging regular bowel movements.

10. Boosts your immune system.
11. Can increase the quantity and quality of your sleep.
12. Gives you better posture, which has a huge impact on your appearance!

What's the best exercise for my face?

Whatever you do you need to enjoy it, and don't over-exert yourself. You might think you are not exercising hard enough, if you have belly fat you can't shift. But because going too hard for too long can raise cortisol levels, it can make you more likely to store fat around your middle.

You need a combination of:

1. Cardio: Every day, if you can, even if it's just a brisk walk or climbing flights of stairs. HIIT gives the biggest growth hormone surge, which is great for skin repair and renewal. However, it's not for the sleep-deprived. Do a minimum of 20 minutes, twice per week.

2. Strength training: 2 to 4 times a week. You can do this with your own body weight, stretchy bands or weights. From the age of 30 we naturally lose 1% of our muscle mass each year, but regular strength training will prevent this. Make sure you get advice: particularly for the right recovery period between workouts for your level of fitness and age, as recovery takes longer as you get older. Back-to-back sessions leave you with inadequate time to repair . . . and that means inflammation. Do legs and arms on alternate days. Also, this may sound obvious, but don't train with injuries. It makes inflammation worse (and it hurts!).

3. Stretching: 2 to 4 times a week, for 30 minutes. Yoga, Pilates and stretching are good for flexibility and joint health. Yoga, my go-to, decreases cortisol and inflammation markers as well as helping balance, strength and being good for weight loss. The moves that involve twisting are good for gut health and elimination. And there's good evidence that yoga puts your body into parasympathetic or relaxation mode, too.

So, is running bad for my face?

NO, not per se. The issue is, people can run too far, too fast, too often. The women who come to the clinic who tell me they use long-distance running as a psychological outlet for stress are often those who go too hard. And intensive training, such as for a marathon, is hard on the face because it leads to loss of fat from all over the body. But it shows dramatically on the face as sagging - which is where the idea of running being bad for your face comes from.

The sag that comes with loss of fat doesn't usually show up until your 40s. At first, as you lose facial fat, you might like the look of sharp cheekbones and jawline. But then, suddenly, you may end up looking drawn and flat, tired or jowly. And this can look more ageing than wrinkles.

If you want to run, follow these rules:

1. Wear sunscreen and a hat. Sunscreen is vital because you're outside, but also sweating increases UV absorption by the skin.
2. Don't over-exert. I see a lot of runners who use running to let off steam, which is going from one stress to another. Take a break of a day or two in between runs! Swap some sessions for yoga or Pilates.
3. Take off your make-up. Make-up blocks sweat and the breakdown products can be very irritating. Cleanse and apply a light moisturizer before any exercise.

CASE STUDY

Treating jogger's face

Kate, 43, is a mum of three. She was pretty stressed and felt miserable when she came into the clinic, not helped by the fact that she thought she looked haggard, from being sleepless and stressed. She told me she was sick of people asking her what was wrong with her. She had booked in for BTX but was prepared to have any treatment to look better. Kate told me that she was running nearly every morning, for an hour or more, using it as her outlet for stress.

The first thing I asked Kate to do was to wear sunscreen and a hat while running. Her skin was very pigmented. I also asked her if she'd consider pausing the running, or at least cutting down. I could tell she didn't want to stop completely, but I explained that she was pushing herself too hard, and so was making her body more stressed. I told her to get more rest, even lying down for 10 minutes during the day and focusing on her breath.

Kate did decide to stop running for a few months. She switched to Pilates and yoga a few times a week and took up strength training in a gym. Crucially she also began to have therapy, so she learnt ways to process her emotions that didn't involve pounding the pavements. She began to have express maintenance facials every 6 weeks (see Chapter 6 for more information on this). After 3 months, she had a minimal amount of BTX, to soften her frown and crows' feet.

Kate has taken up running again, but only a couple of times a week. And she always wears sunscreen and a hat, rain or shine.

On Kate's last visit, she showed me a picture of herself at a wedding 3 years previously. She told me she felt so much better about her looks and in herself. After just 6 months of treatments, she looked both younger and healthier. That was not only down to her skin looking more plump and supple, but she had less pigmentation. And she was a lot less overwhelmed and happier, too.

More effective anti-stress techniques

Choose some of these to add to your daily routine when you have time.

Time in nature

My name for nature is vitamin G, because being surrounded by green has such a powerful anti-stress effect. A growing number of studies show that visiting green spaces and being exposed to natural environments can reduce psychological stress. It's been shown to help with attention fatigue and is linked to increases in self-esteem and mood. Aim for at least 20 minutes of being in nature every day, if you can. Walk or cycle every morning if possible, and go for longer at the weekends. Plan to go the greenest route possible, breathe in the fresh air, and try to switch off and be present in nature.

If you haven't got access to a green space or park, even staring out of the window at the garden or some trees will help, as will investing in some house plants. Not only do plants add vitamin G, they also help purify indoor air, which can be more polluted than outdoors.

Think about the good stuff

There's a proverb from the Hausa tribe that is one of the wisest sayings I've heard: 'Give thanks for a little and you will find a lot.' Keep a journal of the good things that happen to you, small and large. List what you're grateful for, write about someone who was kind to you that day, something you did that made somebody else smile, something you learned. Keep a notepad by your bed to get into the habit of doing this every morning or night - whenever works best for you.

It's worth doing this because the benefits of recognizing what you're grateful for and expressing it include lowered stress and blood pressure, better sleep quality, a stronger immune system and increased feelings of joy, happiness, forgiveness and compassion.

Be with friends

We know that being socially connected is good for our psychological and emotional wellbeing. But studies show that it's vital for physical health too. In fact, a meta-analysis of 70 studies covering over 3 million people showed that not being socially connected actually raises your risk of death. And loneliness has been measured as being as bad for health as obesity and smoking. A lot of us aren't getting enough social contact, even before lockdown. The Office for National Statistics reported that in 2016–17, nearly half (45%) of adults in the UK felt lonely.

First, think about which friendships or relationships, even if they're just with someone you bump into regularly, make you feel good. Are there any groups that leave you feeling happy? Make a list of them. If you can, plan to meet up with these positive people. If you can't see them in person, can you meet them online? Or connect on social media? And is there anything you can give to or do for people in your local community? Numerous studies show that helping others is an excellent wellbeing boost and stress reducer.

Time with you

Get out your diary, as this takes planning. I schedule my personal time into my diary, every day. I do understand that if you're super-busy or you are in the just-trying-to-survive years of having young children, this advice might irk. But you can start with just 5 minutes. That might be your skincare routine. Taking that time for yourself twice a day to carry out this ritual may be the only time of day you get to yourself, to invest in yourself - so take your time and enjoy it.

Now, I've worked up to doing 20 minutes of yoga before everybody gets up. And I never used to take lunch at work, but a walk around the block is my absolute minimum. Every day, I plan a little time to read, to listen to music or even to daydream and do nothing. I try to make sure that chores, like cooking for me, feel more like fun too, by putting on a podcast or allowing my thoughts to wander.

Prioritize your time over what other people want you to do. Here is one of the best pieces of advice a coach ever gave me: to have a No Strategy. He had to tell me this repeatedly over the course of 2 years before I really heard it (you won't hear until you're ready to hear!) - as well as your to-do list, have a not-to-do list - and stick to it.

2. Nutrition

If you've ever looked in the mirror the morning after a big night out, you'll know that what you eat and drink shows up on your skin. This part is about making sure you're getting all the right nutrients for skin health.

Skin, like every organ of the body, needs the correct balance of nutrients. That means carbohydrates for energy, protein for collagen and keratin synthesis, fats for a strong skin barrier and micronutrients for optimal structure and function.

Later in the chapter I will give tips on how to optimize your food choices to support your skin (see 'Eat yourself (more) beautiful', page 84). And I'll also discuss supplements you might need to fill the gaps, due to not having a perfect diet, modern farming methods that lower the levels of nutrients in our foods and your individual genetic make-up.

But I'm going to start with digestion. A healthy digestive system is key because it not only dictates how well you are absorbing the nutrients you eat, but it has a direct influence on the level of inflammation in your body and skin. I've seen some clients with a fantastic diet whose skin just won't behave because of problems in their gut.

That's why I ask new clients about their bowel habits. How often do you go? Any diarrhoea? Constipation? Bloating? Gas? Abdominal pain? If your gut isn't in good shape, you can have the best BTX, you can spend a fortune on skincare, and *still* you won't GLOW.

How to get better gut - and skin - health

I'll go deeper into the skin-digestion connection over the next few pages, but let's begin with a brief overview of the digestive tract, which starts in the mouth and goes all through your body. There are three major issues here that might be affecting your skin.

1. Maldigestion and malabsorption. First, you might not be digesting or absorbing the food you're eating, so your skin isn't getting the nutrients it needs.
2. Gut dysbiosis. This is the name for an imbalance in your gut microbiome (GM), the trillions of bugs that live in your large intestine. When your GM is out of balance, it not only impacts skin nutrient levels but also contributes to inflamm-ageing too.
3. Constipation. Lastly, so many clients I see have constipation, which leads to a build-up of inflammatory toxins in the body.

Now, let's work our way down the digestive tract in more detail . . .

Maldigestion and malabsorption

Mouth

Slow down your eating! Chew each mouthful 20 times. If you're eating food that contains carbohydrates, see how the taste becomes sweeter? This is because of substances called enzymes in your saliva starting to break down the starches into sugars, the first stage of digestion. Chew well and you allow the enzymes to work, making the job easier for your gut later.

Carbohydrates include fruits and vegetables, not just grains and potatoes. If you chew these well, later in the digestive process you're more likely to absorb substances called carotenoids in fruit and veg that are needed for the skin's defence system.

Stomach

The key to the digestion of proteins is having the correct acid level in your stomach. And proteins are the building blocks of healthy skin, hair and nails.

In fact, 40% of people over 40 have significantly low acid levels, known as hypochlorhydria. You can find out about yours by doing this test. First thing in the morning, on an empty stomach, drink ¼ teaspoon of bicarbonate of soda in a small glass of water. If you have sufficient stomach acid levels, within 2 or 3 minutes the alkaline bicarb should react with the acid in your stomach and you'll do a loud belch.

If this doesn't happen, there are acid supplement medications that can help. But it's worth seeing a nutritionist first, especially if you have any other issues with your digestive tract such as bloating or constipation. Adding in more zinc-rich foods, such as oysters, beef, crab (seeds, sea vegetables and wholegrains are vegan alternatives) can also support stomach acid production.

Note: Having to pop an antacid regularly does not mean you have enough acid in your stomach. It can simply mean alcohol or food is sitting in your stomach for too long because it is not broken down.

Small intestine

This is where you absorb the fat from your food. For skin (and whole-body health), it's critical you are not only eating fat (see page 87) but absorbing it. You need to absorb fat so that you can also absorb vitamins A, D, E and K, which all defend skin against the effects of UV damage as well as boosting repair and renewal. These vitamins are 'fat soluble', which means they dissolve in fat and can only be absorbed along with fat.

Vitamin A - also referred to as retinoic acid or retinol - blocks the enzymes (matrix metalloproteinases or MMPs) that break down collagen and elastin when exposed to UV, and stimulates new cell production in the outer epidermis. Found in: eggs, orange and yellow fruit and vegetables.

Vitamin D prevents the skin cell death that's triggered by UVB damage. It also improves repair and the synthesis of new cells at a genetic level. Found in: oily fish (salmon, sardines, mackerel), red meat, egg yolks.

Vitamin E works both superficially to protect against UVB-induced epidermal damage and, deeper in the dermis, helps to protect collagen from its natural tendency to become rigid over time. Found in: nuts and seeds, avocados.

Finally, vitamin K is a potent antioxidant which has been shown to speed up wound healing by stimulating the synthesis of new fibroblasts and improving blood supply. Found in: green leafy vegetables, dairy, beef.

So how can you make sure you're absorbing the fat you need along with these vitamins? Signs that you may not be absorbing it completely are bloating, gas and/or pale, watery stools (this may show they contain undigested fats). Your liver secretes bile to start to break down fats, then your pancreas secretes enzymes to finish the job. Eating bitter leaves, such as chicory (endive), watercress and rocket may help to stimulate digestive enzymes. You can also take a supplement - such as Allergy Research Group 'Full Spectrum Digest' - to support digestion. (If you have any of the above symptoms, it may be a good idea to see a nutritionist.)

Dysbiosis

Gut microbiome (GM) in the large intestine

Your GM is made up of the 100 trillion or so bacteria, viruses, fungi and other microorganisms, good and bad, that live in your gut. They not only further break down food that hasn't yet been digested when it reaches the gut by fermentation, they also have a multitude of other functions, a few of which are explained below.

The overall mix and diversity of the bugs that live in your GM is important and, along with the presence of certain 'bad' bugs (e.g. parasitic infections), has been linked to conditions from acne to obesity to cancer. It's clear that the state of your GM impacts every organ in your body, including your immune system and your skin, although this is an expanding area of research and the exact molecular mechanisms of cross-talk are not fully understood. But what we do know is that a healthy GM is critical.

1. Some vitamins are manufactured by the GM, including some B vitamins. These are one of a multitude of useful by-products of gut fermentation, called postbiotics. Other postbiotics key for skin are vitamins A and K, vitamins I mentioned above.

2. The right balance of gut bugs helps minimize the inflamm-ageing I explained in Chapter 1, which accelerates skin ageing.

One mechanism is via the production of anti-inflammatory postbiotics called short chain fatty acids (SCFA), in particular one called butyrate (also a major source of energy for the gut wall).

3. The functioning of the GM impacts on mood and mental health via many of the body's pathways, including hormones and the immune system, and this is a hot area of research. One of the ways is that it actually produces some key neurotransmitters that directly impact mood, including the feel-good brain chemical serotonin.

How do we know the GM affects skin?

First, disruptions and imbalances to the GM - gut dysbiosis - are almost always seen in inflammatory skin conditions, for example acne, eczema and psoriasis. Second, there is plenty of published data on the beneficial changes in skin quality induced by taking probiotics, supplements that introduce good bugs into your GM. I am always food first when it comes to intervention. But in the 5R approach below, I've also included research on taking daily probiotic supplements to influence the GM because there has been compelling data on their link with skin.

So how do you get more variety in your GM?

There are things you can't control that affect the diversity of your biome, but what you have most control over is what you eat. A boring diet leads to a boring biome, but the good news is that the reverse is true too. Plant polyphenols, chemicals that are abundant in fruits, vegetables, spices and herbs, can instantly boost your biome, as well as being full of antioxidants, anti-inflammatories and soluble fibre, so increasing your intake will start to make a difference straight away. Try to eat as many different ones as possible, as recent research suggests that rather than the traditional 5-a-day that we've been striving for, a more beneficial target is 30 different fruits, vegetables and legumes each week. This way your GM will be able to thrive on a more diverse menu than the same 5 fruit and veg every day.

The 5R approach to GM health

This protocol was designed by the Institute of Functional Medicine (IFM), of which I am a certified member, but has been customized for skin by nutritional therapist Christine Bailey.

1. Remove. The priority is always to follow an anti-inflammatory diet (see page 84, 'Eat yourself (more) beautiful', before starting to cut things out. Then, for one month, avoid or reduce whatever you think you might be eating or drinking to excess, or that might not be helping your gut health. The most common gut irritants are: alcohol, sugar, too much fat, artificial sweeteners or high glycaemic index (GI) foods, which include sugary food but also white carbs. You may know you have other food sensitivities too.

Next steps (under the care of a nutritionist) **could be:**

- Take the probiotic saccharomyces boulardii for one month. Nutritionists use this strong gut bacteria to treat the gut, to encourage it to get rid of parasites, fungi and other bad bugs.
- Or try an elimination diet for 3 weeks (see page 83). As I said, I'm not a fan of restrictive diets, but under the care of a nutritionist this can be an excellent method to determine food intolerances or allergies. Again, designed by the IFM, the diet involves avoiding foods that more commonly cause sensitivity reactions such as gluten grains, dairy, soy, corn, beef, pork, shellfish, peanuts, refined sugars and eggs. And then re-introducing them one at a time, monitoring any gut symptoms.

2. Replace. Support gut motility with added fibre in your diet and replace the factors necessary to optimize digestive secretions, if these are found to be low (again, I recommend seeking the advice of a functional medicine practitioner here). Zinc supplementation may boost stomach acid production, if you are deficient.

3. Repopulate. For long-lasting change in your GM, you need to feed the beneficial bugs in it. You do this by eating particular kinds of dietary fibre that act as their fuel, which is why they are called prebiotics. Soluble fibre is the kind you want, found in root vegetables, oats, rice, bananas, papaya, onions and garlic. Increase your intake gradually, to avoid bloating and cramping. And do not skip this step!

As I've said, my approach to the GM is always food first. So try to include some probiotic foods in your diet. These fermented foods are a great source: kimchi, yoghurt, kefir, sauerkraut and kombucha.

But there's also good research to show that there are beneficial changes in skin quality from taking probiotic supplements, too. For example, multiple studies have shown the impact of specific probiotics on various signs of skin health, such as dermal thickness, hydration and acne breakouts. The probiotic supplement lactobacillus plantarum (LP) was shown to decrease collagen breakdown post UV exposure.

Another probiotic containing bifidobacterium breve helped boost the keratin content of the keratinocytes, the 'bricks' of your epidermis.

Finally, a study showed that taking lactobacillus rhamnosus daily for 12 weeks decreased the expression of IGF-1 in the skin, an inflammatory chemical that promotes excess sebum production and pore clogging in acne.

But do remember that probiotics are like gut tourists - their effect is transient. The aim is more to tweak the environment, so that your own bugs can thrive. If you do want to take probiotics, they are measured in CFU (colony forming units). Look for one that contains at least 20 billion CFU per dose and a mix of strains, so that, again, you're boosting the diversity of your GM.

It's early days, but research is looking into how the skin microbiome - the mix of bugs that live on the skin's surface - changes as the GM changes. There's more about topical probiotic skincare in Chapter 4.

4. **Repair** the lining of the gut. This will optimize nutrient absorption and support your immune system. There's also a really interesting area of research looking at the link between having a healthy gut lining and having a healthy skin barrier.

As I said before, the two surfaces share many similarities, including their function of keeping toxins out. The gut's barrier cells are designed to do just this, but the barrier can break down. This can be due to nutrient deficiencies (for example of zinc or vitamin A), having a poor GM, food intolerances or allergies, excess stress, eating too much sugar, drinking alcohol, and taking certain medications.

When this happens, an inflamed gut lining can allow substances through to the bloodstream that would usually be blocked. This then triggers your immune system to mount an attack on these foreign bodies, and leads to inflammation. This barrier dysfunction is associated with systemic inflammation, as well as many autoimmune diseases and skin conditions such as eczema.

If you suspect this might be an issue, the first step is to look at all the triggers listed above. You can also eat foods rich in micronutrients that can help to heal the gut lining. Meat broths are an excellent source of collagen. This is not only a key protein in the gut lining but also in your dermis, so it supports the skin in two ways. Salad greens are rich in vitamin C, which is vital for new collagen synthesis. Berries contain substances that are believed to inhibit collagen-damaging enzymes (MMPs). Make sure you are eating enough zinc-rich foods too, such as beans, nuts, seafood and dairy, plus foods containing L-glutamine, an amino acid that feeds the cells of the lining and which is found in eggs, fish and poultry.

Also, stop snacking! It's natural to feel hungry between meals. But every time we eat, it triggers an inflammatory response in the gut. Ideally we should eat just 3 times a day, and rest our digestion for 12 hours overnight. But with many of us snacking regularly all day and evening, we keep fuelling the fires of inflammation.

5. **Rebalance**. This step is about rebalancing the GM by reducing your stress levels. The gut is sometimes referred to as a neurological organ, due to its connection to the central nervous system through its rich network of nerves. There is constant feedback between the two, and stress can change the composition of the GM, reducing its diversity. You can tackle stress in all the ways I mentioned in the previous part of this chapter, including deep sleep and regular exercise.

Constipation

You get rid of the body's waste products as well as toxins via your poo. If this isn't happening efficiently, the result might be sallow, spotty skin, or breakouts. It might be that your sweat smells strong. Or it might be wrinkles and sagging, as the circulating toxins cause damage to collagen and elastin fibres.

So how do you know you're eliminating effectively? At the end of the journey through your gut, the aim is to pass one smooth, formed, medium brown stool per day. If you're not doing this, ask yourself the following questions: Am I moving enough? (Exercise helps food move along the gut.) Am I staying hydrated? Am I eating plenty of fruit and vegetables and other plant foods? In particular, am I eating enough soluble fibre? Good sources are: oats, oat bran, rice bran, avocado, apples, peas (see above for more detail).

If you need extra fibre to get things moving, try soaked linseeds or chia seeds. Soak 1-2 teaspoons of cracked linseeds in half a pint of room-temperature water overnight. Drink in the morning, followed by another half pint of water. And then leave 30 minutes before breakfast. Chia seeds are better soaked for 20 minutes (2 tablespoons in 1 cup of water) - then added to smoothies/yoghurt/porridge. If none of that works, try psyllium husk fibre supplements, but take them with plenty of water.

DOES ROSACEA BEGIN IN THE GUT?

In future, we may treat rosacea from the inside out. There's a condition called SIBO, which stands for small intestine bacterial overgrowth, when bacteria of the biome manage to populate the wrong place, that is the small intestine as well as the large. And it's known that SIBO is far more common in rosacea and acne patients - and that treating SIBO has a significant impact on their condition. One study showed that a 10-day course of the antibiotic rifaximin - which cut bacteria in the small intestine - resulted in complete or near eradication of rosacea in 20 out of 28 patients, with significant improvement in a further 6. Results lasted at least 9 months - however, it seems that ongoing treatment is needed. There are alternatives to antibiotics, such as oregano oil and berberine: a functional medicine practitioner can advise you on this.

Eat yourself (more) beautiful

Now you know about absorption of nutrients, which ones should you be getting more of? This isn't about restrictive diet plans because these are often stressful - which we don't want! - and set you up for failure. Instead, I'll suggest skin-supporting foods that you can incorporate into your diet whichever way you like, and supplements that you could consider taking, too.

My super skin eating plan

The most rewarding aspect of changing your diet is eating lots MORE of delicious and nutritious ingredients that are full of skin-friendly ingredients and that will feed your GM and, in turn, make your skin glow. Here's a guide to eating for your skin:

Eat the rainbow, every day

A diverse, plant-based diet will be packed with beneficial fibre and phytochemicals such as polyphenols and other antioxidants to feed your skin and gut - and your general health. That is what makes fruits and vegetables an amazing way to protect your skin from environmental damage as well as ageing. Eating them will lower inflammation levels, improve blood sugar control, and feed your GM. Some of the richest sources are: green tea, apples, cherries and berries, red grapes, red onion, spinach and nuts, as well as dark chocolate and red wine (in moderation!).

The reason why I talk about eating a rainbow is because the benefits often come from the same chemicals that also colour the fruit and vegetables.

- **Red**: Raspberries and pomegranates contain ellagic acid, a polyphenol that blocks release of MMPs, the enzymes that break down collagen when UV hits the skin.
- **Orange**: The lycopene in apricots and papaya (and tomatoes) decreases UV-induced redness. Carotenoids in carrots and cantaloupes are anti-cancer, anti-inflammatory and immune-boosting, as well as decreasing excess sebum production in oily skins.
- **Yellow**: Lemons and pineapples contain bromelain, which is anti-inflammatory.

- **Green**: Watercress boosts your own natural UV protection. Cruciferous vegetables such as broccoli and cauliflower are detoxifiers - especially important for hormone regulation.
- **Purple**: Blueberries are photoprotective, blocking the action of one of the enzymes that breaks down collagen in sunlight.

SOME GOOD SKIN FOODS ARE SURPRISING

Dark chocolate and coffee are also great sources of polyphenols. There are downsides to both, but I think the pros of having them in moderation outweigh the cons. For chocolate, it's the sugar, not the cacao, that's the issue. Cacao is one of the best dietary sources of vitamin A.

Caffeine is an anti-inflammatory and is anti-carcinogenic too. It enhances exercise endurance, mood and clear thinking. It also constricts veins, which helps with flushing. That said, if you have rosacea, hot drinks aren't good, so go for iced coffee.

Coffee's downsides are dependency and sleep disruption, as well as being dehydrating, which is why it's often served with a glass of water in Europe. But it's the sugar and/or the biscuit that often accompanies coffee that really isn't great (see page 89 for more).

Clients ask me whether red wine is a skin food, too. It's not, sorry. This myth came from the fact that it contains resveratrol, a polyphenol from grapes that has been extracted for supplements and used in skincare. It's a long shot to drink wine to access these benefits, and I'm afraid the downsides to alcohol outweigh them.

Eat good fat

As already mentioned, you need fat to absorb vitamins A, D, E and K, which are vital for healthy skin and also for multiple other key functions all over your body. That's why the low-fat diets of the 80s and 90s were - and are - complete nonsense. Let the (extra virgin) olive oil flow! Studies show that it can actually help you to lose weight, decreasing body fat as well as blood pressure. That said, some fats are better than others . . .

EAT MORE: Mono-unsaturated fats (MUFAs) - as they're anti-inflammatory. Good sources are extra virgin olive oil (EVOO), avocados, nuts and seeds.

EAT A GOOD BALANCE: Poly-unsaturated fats (PUFAs). These come in two kinds, omega-3 PUFAs (EPA, DHA and ALA) and omega-6 PUFAs (e.g. linoleic acid), and your body needs both kinds in your diet, as it can't make them itself. But it needs them in a specific proportion. UK guidelines state that 5:1 is the ideal ratio - but some nutritionists say 2:1. Omega-3 is found in particular in oily fish, flax seed and walnuts. Omega-6 is found in raw nuts and seeds, especially sunflower, pumpkin, chia, sesame and hemp and their cold-pressed oils, as well as in grains and refined vegetable oils.

The issue is, most of us don't eat enough omega-3, so our ratio is out. And this ratio is an important indicator of the extent of inflammation in your body. For example, people with acne often have way more omega-6 than omega-3.

You can do a home skin-prick test to find out your ratio. But almost everyone will benefit from an initial reduction in omega-6 PUFAs (abundant in processed foods) and taking an omega-3 supplement.

EAT SOMETIMES: Saturated fats (SFAs). The fats found in butter, dairy and meat have long been seen as bad for you, but this is changing.

Though unhealthy when consumed in excess, SFAs such as butter and ghee are good for higher-temperature cooking, as they don't burn. Coconut oil is also rich in SFAs and appears to be better than animal fats for cooking.

DON'T EAT: Trans fats (TFAs). These are man-made fats that started out as liquid oils but have been processed into a solid. They are used by the food industry for their ability to prolong shelf-life and maintain texture, although they have become less commonly used. TFAs have been linked to unwanted weight gain, inflammation, and an increased risk of several chronic diseases and certain cancers. How do you know to avoid them? Look on the label for 'hydrogenated' or 'partially hydrogenated'.

Eat carbs

Wholegrains are a brilliant source of antioxidants, B vitamins for energy, and magnesium, the anti-stress mineral. Choose wholegrains such as oats, wholegrain rye and millet over high-GI white carbs such as white bread. And choose sweet potatoes, carrots, parsnips and other root vegetables over processed crisps and chips.

Eat herbs and spices

Name something from the spice drawer and you'll likely find it contains skin-friendly phytochemicals. For example, chillies contain a substance that stops collagen breakdown, cinnamon is rich in antioxidants, garlic suppresses pro-inflammatory enzymes. Parsley contains both anti-inflammatories and antioxidants. But the best spice of all is probably turmeric: its anti-inflammatory powers are second to none.

My personal top 10 skin foods

1. Extra virgin olive oil: Anti-inflammatory and helpful for the skin's barrier.
2. Berries: Rich in skin-supporting phytochemicals – antioxidants and anti-inflammatories.

3. Avocados: Full of beneficial fats, mostly MUFAs, as well as vitamins C and E.
4. Brazil nuts: High in MUFAs as well as selenium, an antioxidant mineral.
5. Chia seeds: Good source of fibre, protein and omega-3, as well as zinc for repair.
6. Pomegranates: High in antioxidants. Contain ellagic acid, which reduces UV-induced pigmentation.
7. Sweet potatoes: High in carotenoids, which support skin against UV damage.
8. Watercress: Part of the cruciferous family, a great detoxifier.
9. Salmon: Rich in omega-3, an essential fat.
10. Dark chocolate: Rich in skin and gut-friendly polyphenols.

What to cut out

Sugar

We are all being bio-hacked by the food industry, which has made our taste buds become used to sweeter and sweeter foods. For example, Sainsbury's milk chocolate bar went from 22% sugar in 1992 to 54% in 2019; Cadbury's Dairy Milk jumped from 32% sugar to 55%. The current levels of sugar in our diet - the average is 14 teaspoons per day for UK adults - is WAY higher than nature intended.

But how does all this sugar affect our skin? Glycation, aka 'sugar sag' - a sort of internal caramelization of the skin - is one of the fundamental mechanisms involved in ageing. It's a natural process in which the sugar in your bloodstream attaches to proteins and fats - forming harmful new molecules called 'advanced glycation end products', AGEs for short.

When these accumulate they have been linked to kidney disease, lung disease (COPD) and, more recently, skin ageing. The damage is cumulative and irreversible - rendering skin less firm, more rigid and less elastic.

AGE production is directly related to sugar intake in the diet and is therefore a huge problem for diabetics, where undetected high blood sugar levels can be causing premature ageing for years. Sun exposure also produces AGEs.

What to do?

1. De-normalize sugar! Significantly lowering sugar in your diet for just 4 months has been shown to reduce glycated collagen formation by 25%. After just a week your taste buds will adjust, I promise. You can cut down on obviously sugary foods, and make swaps for others. Swap granola for porridge, sweet popcorn for plain, ice cream for blended frozen bananas, fruit juice for milk or tea, hot chocolate for cocoa, fruit yoghurt for plain yoghurt with chopped fruit.
2. Grilling, roasting, frying and particularly barbecuing create AGEs by caramelizing food. So try to poach, steam or boil instead.
3. Use spices such as cinnamon and cloves, as well as oregano, in cooking to block AGE formation.

Alcohol

Alcohol contributes to and exacerbates all 5 signs of skin ageing, so the best thing to do is keep it to a minimum. That means, at the very least, sticking to the UK Chief Medical Officers' guidelines of 14 units a week, spread over at least 3 days. I'd say stick to a small glass - or two - of wine on the nights you do drink. And have at least 2 days in a row off drinking; 3 is better.

Not convinced? Alcohol dehydrates us massively, which, of course, affects skin hydration levels. It's high in sugar, so contributes to glycation. Drinking also reduces collagen production and antioxidant defences. Plus it directly raises cortisol and oestrogen levels (you want oestrogen, but too much is not a good thing - see page 98) and lowers levels of growth hormone, which is needed for skin renewal.

Finally, excessive drinking destroys facial fat and causes blood vessel dilation on the face, giving that gaunt, ruddy appearance.

How to treat the 5 main signs of facial ageing with diet

To customize the general advice you've just read, the nutrition advice below is specific to the 5 ageing signs. Start by trying one or two changes that sound like they will fit with your lifestyle. You don't have to do everything at once!

Dull, dry complexion

To speed slow cell renewal, eat more plant polyphenols to upregulate cell renewal genes (see Eat the rainbow, page 85).
To strengthen your skin barrier, boost your PUFA intake to boost the skin's lipid matrix. It might be worth investing in omega-3 supplements. It's found in fish oil but also in vegan supplements (Nuique is a good brand).

The omega-6 fatty acid GLA also helps prevent water evaporation from the skin. You'll find this in evening primrose oil, and borage seed oil supplements. (Don't take omega-6 without omega-3 - see page 87 for why.)

You could also try L-histidine supplements, which boost the production of filaggrin, an essential building block of the skin's barrier. They've been shown to have the same efficacy as steroids in the treatment of atopic dermatitis.

Red, sensitive skin

Follow the advice for a weak skin barrier, as above. In particular eat the rainbow and take omega-3. Plus, keep to low glycaemic foods. The general rule is, no sugar and no processed or white carbs. Also eat foods rich in vitamin D (oily fish, mushrooms, egg yolk) and vitamin A (eggs, liver).

Avoid foods high in toxic metals (arsenic, lead, mercury) from the environment, such as tuna and swordfish, as well as foods containing artificial additives, and trans fats. Experiment with cutting out foods that may be causing an inflammatory reaction. This might be red meat, dairy, or members of the nightshade family such as peppers and aubergines. See page 80 for my guidelines on the elimination diet. However, if you are cutting out a food group, do this under the advice of a nutritionist.

Pigmentation

Increase your intake of vitamin C. You can also eat pomegranates and/or drink pomegranate juice; these contain ellagic acid, which suppresses the production of melanin. Additionally, supplements containing the antioxidant pycnogenol, an extract of pine bark, have been shown to treat the brown blotches of melasma.

Wrinkles

Eating plants that are rich in carotenoids, such as spinach which contains lutein, will boost your natural defences to UV rays. In fact, eating more polyphenols of all kinds is great for skin (see page 85 for more sources). Cocoa and green tea have both been shown to reduce or protect against the effects of MMPs, the enzymes that break down collagen and elastin.

Sagging

Avoid sugar and high GI foods. The process of glycation makes collagen fibres rigid, and also extremely difficult for your body to repair or replace. More severe sagging is caused by both fat and bone loss that happen naturally with age, in the lower face in particular.

Bone loss accelerates after the menopause, so see page 96 for advice on hormones.

Which supplements are best for skin?

In an ideal world we would be getting all our nutrients from the food we eat, but that is an almost impossible task these days, for two reasons.

First, we live fast-paced lives that don't allow us to cook from scratch and forage the best herbs and spices every day. Also our food choices may be cutting our sources of nutrition too. We don't eat as much liver, an excellent source of zinc, vitamin A and selenium. People following a vegan diet can be low in calcium, iron and vitamin B12 if they don't plan food carefully. The National Diet and Nutrition Survey sadly confirms that most of us don't eat 5 fruits and vegetables a day, or enough oily fish, and certainly not the 30 different plant-based foods per week that we should really be hitting.

Second, our food is not as rich in nutrients as it used to be. This is mainly due to farming practices changing the soil quality, but also a lot of our fruit and vegetables are being modified to taste less bitter, and the essential antioxidants are what give these foods their bitterness.

So that's where supplements come in . . .

The 'one-size-fits-all' diet does not exist; each of us has individual biochemical needs. And the Recommended Daily Amounts you'll see on supplement bottles may help to prevent the classic deficiency diseases (such as rickets and scurvy, caused by vitamin D and C deficiencies), but they are really too low to be used as targets for optimal health.

And there are now tests which identify a whole host of genetic variants that show you may need higher doses of vitamins and minerals than other people to function optimally. At the clinic, we use HumanPeople, a leading specialist in precision nutrition. Not only do they test for the genetic variants mentioned above, but they also layer in additional data by testing your blood and gut microbiome. By taking such a holistic and individualized approach, they are able to provide the precise combination of high-quality supplements proven to make a difference for optimum health. Each month they send out a box of daily supplement packs, uniquely tailored to you and reviewed (at-home testing) every 3 months.

However, there are some supplements which will likely benefit almost everyone's skin. These are my top 7:

1. Omega-3. Look for a combination of over 700mg DHA/EPA. Try: Minomi. In a study of 3,000 people, those with higher levels of omega-3 in their diet had a lower rate of sun-induced ageing.
2. Vitamin D3 PLUS K2. Take 2-4,000U per day - the higher dose in winter, as that's when we're most likely to be deficient. For best absorption, take one that contains vitamin K2, plus calcium if you're vegan. You can usually get your vitamin D levels tested if you ask your GP, otherwise you can do it privately for around £36.
3. Vitamin C. Take 1,000mg per day. As well as being a potent antioxidant and protecting your skin from UV damage, vitamin C is essential for fibroblasts to make collagen, and the production of cholesterol and ceramides for a strong skin barrier. Best for skin if taken in combination with vitamin E.
4. Magnesium. Take magnesium glycinate, 200mg per day. Boosts skin hydration by improving barrier function, reduces skin roughness and inflammation. It will also help with stress and sleep. If you are having trouble sleeping, try taking the above twice a day for 2 weeks to see if that helps.
5. Zinc. Take 15mg per day. The World Health Organization estimates that 30% of the global population are deficient in zinc. And mild zinc deficiency can lead to rough, dehydrated skin and impaired wound healing.

6. Probiotics for gut heath (take as described on page 81). Look for one that contains at least 20 billion CFU per dose and a mix of strains.
7. Astaxanthin. Take 7mg per day. This is a type of carotenoid that causes the pink colour of salmon, trout and prawns. It's a great antioxidant and anti-inflammatory and helps support collagen repair, blocking its breakdown.

COLLAGEN SUPPLEMENTS: ARE THEY WORTH THE HYPE?

Collagen supplements are all the rage at the moment - particularly within the skinfluencer community. The idea is, when you take them, the building blocks of collagen flood the system and trick the body into thinking it has to repair and regenerate. But the data isn't there yet. Whether the collagen you take leads to more collagen in the skin, I'm not 100% convinced. So yes, it might be worth doing, but don't hang all your hopes on it and don't squeeze yourself financially to have this on your shelf. It would be much better to invest in a combination of the above.

Acne and diet

Studies show a definite link between diet and acne, although it might not be the one you think. People assume that chocolate is the culprit. But in fact all high GI foods, including sugary foods but also white bread, white rice and potatoes, seem to exacerbate acne. There's also a weak association between eating dairy and acne, although I'd recommend seeing a nutritionist to help guide you through excluding any food.

DRINK UP!

I mean green tea . . . This is power hydration, packed with polyphenols, antioxidant-rich, anti-carcinogenic, and it contains tons of vitamins C and E. I drink 3 cups a day, sometimes hot and sometimes cold, with a twist of lemon to boost antioxidant absorption.

3. Hormones

There is so much more to hormones than sex and fertility. Hormones are the body's little messengers, traffic lights controlling all systems from urinary and respiratory to digestive and muscular. They dictate and regulate so much of what we feel: tired, hot, hungry and, of course, horny.

Produced by glands around the body - the thyroid, adrenal, pituitary, as well as the ovaries and testes - hormones are circulated through the bloodstream to make their mark on the structure and function of tissues and organs. When they go out of balance, which is often during periods of stress or at certain life stages (puberty, menopause, old age), this can start a cascade of problems, from infections and insatiable cravings to infertility, disease, and what we are going to discuss here, skin issues and accelerated ageing.

The more out of balance your hormones are, the faster you will age. The good news is they aren't out of our control. Although it's an incredibly complex area, there are lifestyle changes you can make to help keep your hormones under control.

Key hormones for skin

All hormones play vital roles in our bodies, so you can't say they are either good or bad, heroes or villains. But there are some that can really make a difference to how fast you age. They include cortisol, which I've explained in the Stress section (see page 55). As you already know, sustained high levels of cortisol accelerate every one of the 5 age-related skin concerns, in particular reduced elastin and collagen and production of lipids in the barrier layer, leading to thinner, weaker, dehydrated skin.

In this section, I'll explain the effects of some other key hormones, including oestrogen, DHEA, growth hormone and thyroid hormones, on skin and health. I'll also describe key ways to get them into balance, so you'll feel and see the difference. Here's a rundown on getting your hormones working for you.

The sugar hormone: insulin

Insulin's function is to lower blood sugar levels. The trouble comes when levels of insulin peak and stay too high because of our sugary diets. Then, too much insulin reduces the activity of growth hormone (see page 101) because they both compete for the same receptors.

Persistently high sugar levels can also lead to insulin resistance, when the body stops responding to insulin. And insulin production also naturally declines with age. The result of both of these is rising sugar levels in the blood. As I explained above, as sugar levels rise, your skin begins to caramelize in a process called glycation, becoming thin and rigid, which I've described above as 'sugar sag' (see page 89).

To maintain a healthy level of insulin in your system, try to cut out sugar as well as high GI foods, which are foods that make blood sugar levels go up fast, after you eat them. Make sure you get enough sleep and regular exercise, which also helps with insulin control (see page 69).

The glow hormone: oestrogen

Oestrogen is the most important hormone - for women - for looking and feeling good. It's a big player in skin health, involved in barrier function, collagen production, skin hydration and thickness. It also improves wound healing. When oestrogen is high - such as during pregnancy - it can reduce the symptoms of psoriasis.

Oestrogen is produced in the ovaries but also, in a weaker form, by the adrenal glands and fat cells. And importantly, like all hormones, it's a balancing act; both too much and too little are bad, triggering an inflammatory response.

Too much: oestrogen dominance

This means too much oestrogen relative to the other main female hormone, progesterone, which is essential for skin elasticity. Oestrogen dominance can present as a wide range of symptoms, from heavy, painful and irregular periods to breast tenderness, fatigue, depression and anxiety. It is often a factor in PMS, fibroids and endometriosis.

Being overweight can compound the situation because fat cells produce oestrogen too. Another factor is the effect of substances called xenooestrogens. These are oestrogen mimickers or 'dirty' oestrogens in your diet and environment. They bind to and block oestrogen receptors, increasing levels of circulating oestrogen. They're found in pesticides, exhaust fumes, bisphenol A (a plastics additive), cigarette smoke, grilled meat, milk, water and cosmetics. We are ALL exposed every day!

As your body's detoxification pathways go into overdrive to break down all the excess oestrogen, you end up with a build-up of harmful oestrogen breakdown products. One way to help eliminate these is to eat cruciferous vegetables every day, such as broccoli, cabbage, kale and Brussels sprouts.

Too little: perimenopause and menopause

Your production of oestrogen can become erratic from as early as your 30s, with surges of high levels alternating with periods of low levels. These hormonal imbalances can start a long time before a blood test at your GP will confirm changes.

However, the most common age for women to really notice symptoms from dropping oestrogen is the mid to late 40s. This is called the perimenopause, as you are only considered to be officially menopausal after you haven't had a period for a full year.

There are oestrogen receptors in nearly all the tissues of the body, so symptoms of fluctuating or low oestrogen are wide-ranging too, including hot flushes, brain fog, lower sex drive, tiredness and vaginal dryness and mood changes, as well as irregular periods. In the skin, low oestrogen shows up as dry skin and a sharp fall in plumpness and radiance.

Signs of facial ageing are linked to how long you have been oestrogen deficient rather than your age. Collagen levels decrease 30% in the first 5 years of menopause. Some women choose to take HRT (hormone replacement therapy), which is most commonly oestrogen and progesterone. Taking HRT for 12 months has been proven to improve epidermal hydration, dermal thickness and elasticity as well as improving collagen quality and skin blood supply, and so fewer wrinkles.

I have seen the difference that HRT can make to skin as well as to all the other symptoms of menopause. But it's not my place to advise you on whether to take it; it's such a personal decision. One thing I will say - the benefits to both mind, body and skin make it worth real consideration. Do at least research it with the help of your GP or gynaecologist, then you can make an educated decision.

Research shows that high stress can exacerbate menopause symptoms. Exercise, sleep and cutting down on alcohol are key, as is eating the diet recommended above. You could also try adding sources of phytoestrogens, which help balance oestrogen. These include soy, flax seeds and pulses, chickpeas, alfalfa, peanuts and supplements such as red clover. These will help mitigate skin ageing caused by falling oestrogen levels and could help with other menopausal symptoms, too (though do not take in excess if you have a hormone-related cancer).

Get more information on menopause health via the Balance App and themenopausedoctor.co.uk.

Dehydroepiandrosterone (DHEA)

This is the mother hormone, made by the adrenal glands and converted into both oestrogen and testosterone. Levels start to come down from the age of 35 years. Stress will often make this worse: if you are often stressed, you'll be asking your adrenals to produce stress hormones, rather than do their other jobs.

DHEA becomes more important when production of oestrogen starts to reduce during perimenopause. Some practitioners recommend taking DHEA supplements. I'd say be very cautious indeed and take them under expert supervision, because they can boost *all* hormone levels, including that of cortisol.

A word on adrenal fatigue. This is the result of prolonged exposure to mental, emotional or physical stress. It's when the adrenal glands are constantly producing cortisol in response to stress, and this eventually leads to adrenal 'burn-out' and a permanent low cortisol state. This might sound positive, but you do need some cortisol.

At its most serious, adrenal fatigue can show up as panic attacks, weight gain (particularly around your stomach), a poor libido and, when your cortisol flatlines, burn-out. The way to tackle adrenal fatigue long-term is rest, sleep, gentle exercise and stress management. One useful supplement is rhodiola, but if you are worried about tiredness, you might want to see your GP or a functional medicine practitioner, as there are lots of potential causes.

Growth hormones

The growth hormones - HGH and IGF-1 - are all about growth, repair, regeneration and building new cells. They stimulate collagen production and cell turnover and renewal. Growth hormone deficiency leads to sagging, so you definitely want more of these!

Sadly, levels fall even from your 20s. By your 60s, you're producing 80% less than you did as a teenager. Sleep is a critical factor here - by the age of 30 most of us will only make GH when in deep sleep. All the other elements of good lifestyle are key too, in particular a low sugar and low GI diet. When you exercise, do HIIT if you can, and definitely strength training. Smoking in particular is terrible for HGH levels, so if you smoke, give up. And sex is extremely good, as is masturbation.

Thyroid hormones

These hormones, produced by a gland in the front of the neck, are involved in regulating nearly every organ in the body. They stimulate different metabolic functions in the cells, help us grow hair, give us energy, regulate our temperature and weight, balance our blood sugar, hydrate our skin, and much more.

The high cortisol that comes from stress reduces thyroid hormone levels. And having low thyroid hormones (called hypothyroidism) can result in dry, thin skin, eye bags, and puffiness due to fluid retention. High levels of thyroid hormones can show up as itchy skin, flushing and thinning hair. Ask your GP for a test if you have any concerns.

How to rebalance your hormones

All the advice in the Stress section earlier in the chapter (see page 55) is beneficial for your hormones as well as for your skin. But if you think that you could benefit from some support to your hormone balance, add in the following advice that's more specific, too:

1. Reduce toxins from your diet and environment. Smoking in particular will have an effect on your thyroid, as will intake of the xenooestrogens, the oestrogen-mimickers that come from the environment (see page 98 for more).
2. Boost your hormone detoxification. Vegetables in the cruciferous family contain substances that bind to oestrogen metabolites as well as other toxins and so help you excrete them. The active ingredient, an extract called DIM (diindolylmethane) is also available as a supplement. Other foods to eat are: onions, garlic, turmeric, herbs and avocado. Another detoxification supplement is NAC (N-acetylcysteine), which helps support the liver - take 400-800mg daily.
3. Eat high-quality protein on a daily basis, essential for building the enzymes and transporters required for hormone metabolism. Wild fish, poultry, eggs, pea protein powder and a little lean meat will also provide vitamins B6 and B12, important for hormone detoxification pathways.
4. Have sex. It's age-defying on so many levels. There are so many benefits triggered by touch alone, with a whole host of hormones released that help to relieve stress, including beta-endorphin; a natural opiate, prolactin, which gives the post-coital 'aah', and oxytocin which drives feelings of affection. All three are released during orgasm - giving the high but also the benefit of post-coital slumber - that deep sleep our body craves. During sex, blood flow increases to all the organs, including skin. And sweat also has skin-

softening oils, which accounts for the post-coitus afterglow. It doesn't have to be sex - masturbation, cuddling and kissing are all good too, boosting circulation, increasing immunity, and decreasing your risk of heart disease. And if sex isn't on the menu, you can still get oxytocin release from a cuddle or hug with a friend, family member or your children.

4. Environment

The news that the environment you live in affects your skin is not new. I must have given the advice to wear sunscreen thousands of times in clinic (and more than once in this book!).

But I still hear so much resistance to it. Sunscreen really is the number one skin-changer, over time. A huge 80% of the signs of facial ageing can be attributed to sun exposure. And as you know, UV damage is the leading cause of skin cancer, too.

That's one reason I've put the environment at this low, key level of the PAP. We need to protect our skin from outer attack. The other factors affecting your skin from outside are smoking (you probably also know this is terrible for skin - but I want to underline that), and pollution, where research is new and growing.

The UV spectrum

UVB rays cause sunburn and are particularly active when the sun shines. But UVA rays are hitting your skin every day, even when it rains. They pass through glass - your windscreen and windows - and they penetrate 40 times deeper into the skin, deep into the dermis, destroying the collagen and elastin fibres that are the building blocks of your skin, causing uneven pigmentation and DNA mutations.

Here's the damage they're both doing at a cellular level:

- UVB rays cause immune system havoc - a single episode of sunburn can suppress your immune system for 2 weeks. They also cause DNA mutations, which can lead to skin cancer.
- UVA rays raise the skin's levels of free radicals, which attack the structure of skin on many levels: proteins such as collagen and elastin, membrane lipids and DNA. They also induce micro-tearing of collagen fibres.

But there is good news: it's never too late to start wearing sunscreen. In fact, one study found that daily sunscreen can actually reverse signs of ageing.

When it comes to darker skin tones, sunscreen is still vital. Differences in skin tones come down to the size and distribution of pigment within melanocytes (the cells that produce the dark pigment melanin), which is why reactions to and healing times from treatments can vary with skin tone. However, *all* skin tones need sunscreen. The ingredients that both benefit skin and are a problem for skin are global, regardless of race or heritage.

If we look again at the top 5 ageing signs I see in the clinic, we can see how exposure to the sun can affect every single one:

Dry, dull complexion

Because UV exposure thickens the epidermis, it gives skin that leathery, weatherbeaten appearance.

Redness/sensitivity

UV rays induce a massive inflammatory response. And inflammation has a knock-on effect on lots of issues. For instance, 80% of rosacea is thought to be down to UV exposure.

Pigmentation

The sun is the number one cause of pigmentation. And as you get older, you're more prone to uneven pigmentation. One study showed that this can add up to 10 years to the perceived age of your face.

Wrinkles

The inflammatory response to UV rays boosts your skin's production of collagen-degrading enzymes, triggering collagen breakdown. UV also reduces new collagen synthesis.

Sagging

UV exposure leads to elastosis, a drop in elastin quality and production and so a loss of spring and elasticity in the skin.

I'll discuss which sunscreens to use in more detail in Chapter 4, but the most important thing of all is to avoid the sun. Please sit in the shade and wear a hat and glasses as often as you can.

Should we worry about blue light?

Blue light is part of the visible light spectrum. It's early days for research, but it has been shown to generate free radicals. That's why there's been lots of noise in the media recently about the blue light emitted by the devices we use on a daily basis, such as the phone and PC, ageing our skin. However, my feeling is that we still get more blue from visible light exposure than we do from devices.

And although iron oxide has been touted as a new and important protective skincare ingredient, blocking visible light in the blue range, a good broad spectrum sunscreen should suffice. When science throws out something interesting, often marketeers spin it out when the research is still too thin. This seems to be the case here - it's marketing hype!

Sunscreen and vitamin D

You have probably heard of vitamin D's importance for healthy bones, but it's also vital for the proper function of nearly every tissue in our bodies, including our brain, heart, muscles, immune system and skin. Vitamin D deficiency has been linked to a wide range of skin diseases and disorders, including acne, rosacea, psoriasis and even skin cancer. And most people in the UK are deficient in it.

You may also have read that it's the action of UV on our skin that helps us produce vitamin D. That's why it's sometimes called the sunshine vitamin. Some people use this as an argument against wearing sunscreen, or for leaving the skin bare for a certain period every day. It's true that daily sunscreen use does indeed reduce vitamin D production. But having seen the damage that UV does to skin, my advice is still to apply sunscreen to your face, every day. You can get some vitamin D from foods - such as oily fish (salmon, mackerel, sardines), liver, red meat and egg yolks. But, to get enough and to save your face, take a supplement (see page 94 for details).

SKIN CANCER

Around 15,400 people are diagnosed with melanoma in the UK each year and the rates are rising. In fact, the incidence of malignant melanoma in Britain has risen faster than any other common cancer. Since 1997 there has been an increase of 155% for over-55s and 63% for under-55s.

If you have a family history of skin cancer you'll certainly be more susceptible and should absolutely take more care to avoid UVA rays. Sunbeds are a huge risk factor, but so too is a history of blistering sunburn in your childhood; the more often this happened, the greater the risk. Which means that pretty much all of us need regular mole screening and full-body check-ups. Don't put it off.

Smoking

It goes without saying that no one should smoke. Never mind the impact it has on your skin health, your overall health will seriously suffer if you continue.

There are strong links between smoking and squamous cell carcinoma (skin cancer), psoriasis, poor wound healing, and diabetic skin lesions. It also makes hair go grey earlier and contributes to hormone-related hair loss (androgenic alopecia).

The term 'smoker's face' is used to sum up the many signs of premature skin ageing that smoking causes: lots of wrinkles, either an ashen, pale complexion or a flushed, red one, and/or a face that's puffy or gaunt.

But how does this happen? There are multiple ways smoking destroys skin. The nicotine makes you pee more, so your skin dehydrates. Your collagen breaks down faster. Your skin's vitamin A levels plummet. Blood flow to the skin goes down, decreasing the supply of nutrients and oxygen, encouraging a build-up of toxic waste products and resulting in a reduced ability to heal.

Genes are important here, as women and people who have lighter skin tones are more affected. But whatever your genes, someone who's smoked a pack a day for 50 years will be on average nearly 5 times more wrinkled than a non-smoker. Even after 8 years of smoking one pack per day - you'll have significantly more wrinkles.

Pollution

In modern life, we are surrounded by pollution in various forms, from exhaust fumes to air-conditioning and carpet hairs. It's a relatively new area of research, but studies show a definite link between airborne pollutants and signs of facial ageing – in particular pigmentation and wrinkles. One study showed an increased prevalence of acne due to higher sebum production. Other studies showed that pollutant particles from traffic were associated with an increase in age-related brown spots on the forehead and cheeks, and an increase in wrinkles and skin laxity.

What might be the mechanisms at play?

Pollution has been shown to disturb the skin microbiome, therefore weakening its defence to unfriendly microbes, and to break down barrier lipids, leading to dehydration and dryness.

Pollution also activates inflammatory pathways, increasing the damaging free radicals I described in Chapter 1 (page 17), and decreasing levels of antioxidants.

Interestingly, the make-up of the skin microbiome seems to have an influence on the impact of pollution, posing the question: could changing this be useful in preventing pollution's ageing effects? For now, try to get more fresh air if and when you can, and eat the antioxidant-rich diet suggested on page 85.

CHAPTER ROUND-UP

- Sun, sugar and smoking are traditionally the big NO-NOs for ageing skin – but the opportunity to influence the ageing process does not stop here.

- The adjustments that really work fall into 4 categories: diet and good gut health; stress management; balancing your hormones; and boosting your environmental defences.
- Eat a diverse, plant-based diet, to support your gut biome. Eat the rainbow.
- Monitor and address symptoms of poor gut health (belching, abdominal pain, flatulence, constipation or diarrhoea). Problems in your gut will likely end up showing on your skin.
- Do not underestimate the negative effect of stress - it can cancel out ALL the benefits of a stellar diet.
- A good lifestyle will go a long way to helping keep your hormones balanced. But if that isn't enough, do see your GP.
- As you get older, what will count the most is good sleep, regular exercise and feeling connected to friends, family and community. These have an enormous impact on your health, inside and out.

Chapter Four

Active skincare

Although people often come to me for aesthetic procedures, I am actually most enthusiastic about skincare. Yes, you have to be realistic, and, yes, there is only so much you can achieve with skincare alone when addressing certain issues. But, armed with the right knowledge, the right ingredients and a consistent routine, you really can achieve quite unbelievable results.

When I first started to practise, my passion for skincare would often take over and I'd bombard clients with all my knowledge at once. Most had come to me for quick fixes and so they'd leave the surgery feeling completely overwhelmed and even more wedded to the sensory highs of binge-purchasing in beauty halls, or the simplicity and ease of soap and water.

Now my approach is much simpler. It's about taking small steps that slowly improve the function of your skin, not just improving the cosmetic impact. You will glow now, yes, but at the same time you'll also be investing in maintenance and prevention. And you can do most of this yourself at home, no clinic required.

In this chapter, I will set out my skincare guidelines, and show you where to start with your new routine. And, of course, I will throw in some myth-busting to help you cut through the noise and hype of the skincare companies. As exciting as all those product launches may seem, you'll discover that it's correct and consistent use of the few maximal strength active ingredients that are right for you that works best.

I call my approach active skincare, because I use biologically active, targeted ingredients that change skin structure and function. My favourite three are: vitamin A, vitamin C and acid exfoliators, as well as a whole range of other add-on ingredients.

People are often nervous of active ingredients or more highly concentrated formulations, or unsure how to use them. But once you start using active skincare, you'll start to see results. That might be calming your skin, strengthening it, even preventing ageing - as well as a cosmetic upgrade. Used with care and the knowledge and expertise I'm going to share, you'll find it can be truly transformative.

The rules for success

I'm going to explain my key rules first, then go into them in detail along with programmes to suit your skin issue. My approach to each one is based both on the science of skin and skincare, and on what I've seen works best on clients in the clinic.

Results won't be instant - indeed, most of the programmes are at least 3 months, although you'll see changes earlier. So what are the signs you'll see when your skincare is really working for your skin?

You'll wear less make-up. Don't get me wrong, I love make-up. But it's wonderful to have the choice not to wear it, to enjoy leaving the house make-up free as well as experimenting when you feel like it.

You won't need a thick, gloopy moisturizer. You might be surprised to learn that you don't need to use a thick moisturizer. Certainly if you're in your 30s and 40s, needing this kind of moisturizer is an indicator that your skin barrier is in a less than optimal state and you're using moisturizer to compensate. I'll help you get your skin into optimal condition, so it will become better at sealing in its own moisture and preventing irritants from entry.

You won't need to go to a clinic. Once again, don't get me wrong, I love my BTX and fillers! But injectables alone don't often give someone that 'wow' factor. Having good skin means you're less likely to want treatments, and if you do choose to have them, they'll continue to look good and will even seem to last longer. You may not feel so desperate as the effects wear off and you're less likely to come to rely on them - so you'll be able to avoid the tell-tale signs of having had treatment well into your 60s plus.

Rule 1: Keep it simple

You don't need a complicated 10-step regime to see fantastic results. When it comes to skincare, less can be so much more. Although it can take a while to get there, once your skin is functioning optimally you really can have a 4-step maintenance regime. That said, there is no magic bullet to your ideal skin, and you will need a range of products, not just soap and water.

Or perhaps you're one of the people who loves the multi-layered approach? If that's you, if you have the time and enjoy spending it on your skincare 'ritual', you can build up from my super-simple regime to a multi-layered approach.

Whatever your routine is now, I'll teach you how to start your new routine with the 5 skincare BASICS that every skin needs: sunscreen, cleanser, vitamin A, acid exfoliant, antioxidant serum. From that base, you can then layer up with TARGETED add-on ingredients if and when you need or want them.

However, do not confuse the basics as being either *low maintenance* or *zero commitment*! For any skincare regime to work – whether it's 4-step or 10-step – you will need to commit your time (daily and long-term) and some of your budget to see results.

While I am all about simplicity and I will always be a low-maintenance woman at heart, unfortunately the older you get the more time and money you have to commit to achieve results. That said, there are products that are less expensive and very good, and products that cost hundreds of pounds where you're simply paying for the brand and the marketing, not the actual effectiveness of the product. In this chapter, I'll explain the brands I recommend, usually both because they have the science to back them up and because I've seen them get results.

Rule 2: Do no harm

Stop the quick fixes! When it comes to skincare, as with so many things in life, it's a marathon, not a sprint. Consistency and patience will win every time.

What I've seen so often is a constant and sporadic search for quick fixes leading to inflammation. People chop and change their products in their search for what works. This reduces our healing capacity, weakens the skin barrier, making it more permeable, and ultimately accelerates the breakdown of collagen and elastin in the deeper layers. Which we then try and fix with more products . . .

That's why you might think your skin is 'sensitive'. But we *all* have sensitive skin. It's one of our skin's roles to sense, alert us and adapt.

What your skin probably really is, is sensitized. One reason might be that you're using the wrong products for your skin type, or for your skin concern. Because these are different things. Your skin type is your 'tendency' to have oiliness, pigmentation, wrinkling, dry or sensitive skin. This is dictated by your genetics.

On that note, skin of colour is not a skin type per se. Fitzpatrick Skin Typing classifies skin into 6 types, according to the amount of melanin skin contains (see page 21 for an explanation of melanin). However, higher levels of melanin in darker skin make it more prone to pigmentation when triggered, for example after a spot or trauma. And a lower concentration of ceramides in the barrier layer gives darker skin a tendency to increased moisture loss and so to dryness.

Your Fitzpatrick type is not nearly as important as whether your skin is dry or oily when choosing your skincare regime. And skincare needs to change to suit skin condition, a snapshot of skin's current status. As we know from Chapter 3, diet, environment, lifestyle and hormonal imbalance can turn your skin type upside down; nothing's set in stone!

For example, in winter, lower humidity makes many of us prone to dryness. And extremes of temperature (cold outside, central heating inside) will make those skins that are genetically prone to redness and sensitivity likely to flare up.

Later in the chapter, I'm going to explain more about how this sensitivity happens, and how to break the cycle and get it into its best-ever condition.

You'll see that I always start people off on their skin programme by going back to the 5 BASICS. You may miss all your different products, but once you see how good your skin looks, you won't. And once your skin has healed, you may be able to add them - or some of them - back in.

Rule 3: Pay attention

You know your skin better than anyone, so pay attention to it. There are so many things that influence our skin from day to day and month to month, from the products you are using, to your menstrual cycle, to your diet, as well as the seasons. Then there are life events, such as pregnancy, stress and generally getting older. Note any changes, then respond gently and with care.

On page 160 you'll find a quiz you can take before, during and after your new skincare regime. When it comes to skincare, if in doubt, always go back to the 5 key BASICS. I'll explain more about how to do this later in the chapter.

Rule 1: Keep it simple

Skincare basics

Finding your 5 key basics, AKA the stuff that really does work, is the key to Rule 1: Keep it simple. Get them right, and they are the best foundation for great skin.

The basics have two functions. The first is to support and boost your natural defences. And the key products to do this are sunscreen and cleanser, as well as moisturizer. The second is to boost your skin's natural repair and regenerative processes. These are the three As: acid exfoliants, antioxidants, such as vitamin C, and vitamin A (also called retinoids).

A.M.	P.M.
Cleanser	Cleanser
Antioxidant serum	Acid exfoliant +/or vitamin A*
Moisturizer (if needed)	Moisturizer (if needed)
Sunscreen	

Looking at the table, you'll see you have 7 or 8 steps to complete with 5 or 6 products. I've put a star next to acid exfoliant and vitamin A because, as I explain later, you might not use both or either every day.

And, as I'll also explain later, you may end up not needing moisturizer at all.

Below are the basics. I've put them in order of priority, rather than the order you apply them.

Basic 1: The boss - sunscreen

If you've read the first few chapters of this book, you know how I feel about sunscreen! I've put it first because it really is the most essential part of your morning routine. There are now so many to choose from on the market at a range of prices, but these are the key points:

Use SPF50 if you can - but SPF30 will do. I say this because there is officially only a 1% difference in protection level, if you use enough. And enough is half a teaspoon, covering your neck and lips too. The sunscreen you choose - the one you can use regularly - will depend on how the product feels on your skin. The higher factors tend to have a thicker, greasier texture, making them harder to apply well and not as nice to wear. So if you find a SPF30 you love and therefore are happy to use every day, that will do just perfectly!

As you may know, there are two types of sunscreen ingredient. The first is physical (also called mineral and inorganic), made up from tiny particles of zinc oxide or titanium dioxide. The second is chemical (confusingly, also called organic). There's debate about which one to use, and it's difficult to give clear-cut advice on this. And some products are a combination of the two.

The 'more natural' campaigns will tell you to use physical sunscreens - but in fact all sunscreens are full of chemicals. There's also a myth that physical sunscreens reflect light, and chemical ones absorb it, which heats up the skin. That's why some people think their pigmentation is made worse by chemical sunscreens. In fact, both work in the same way, by absorbing UV and converting it to heat. Physical sunscreens reflect 10% of UV, at the most.

Some people find the white cast of physical sunscreens off-putting, as well as the thicker texture. If you find them too heavy or you've found they make you break out, there are lighter-textured versions now, such as Avène Mineral Fluid, SPF50.

Chemical sunscreens can give you higher protection, especially from UVA light. They have lighter textures, no white cast, and stay put better. But they can be more irritating for some people.

Chemical sunscreens are also much harder to remove. Which is important, as I believe a build-up of sunscreen over days/weeks is what causes many sensitivity issues. Avoid these ingredients if you find your skin is sensitized by sunscreen: octocrylene, oxybenzone, avobenzone, PABA. Generally, physical sunscreens can be better for sensitive skins.

My advice is to find a sunscreen you are comfortable wearing every day. But whichever one you choose, be sure to cleanse thoroughly at night.

If you are indoors all day, you don't need to wear the same sunscreen you would on the beach, and you don't need to keep reapplying it. But remember, UVA penetrates glass. Medik8 Advanced Day Total Protect SPF30 is good for non-beach days.

Two good physical sunscreens are: Neostrata Sheer Physical Protection SPF50 and REN Clean Screen Mineral SPF 30.

For chemical sunscreens, look for the ingredients Mexoryl XL and Tinosorb M, which protect against both UVA and UVB. Try: Avène Suncare Cream SPF50. La Roche-Posay Anthelios XL SPF 50+ Ultra-Light Fluid is a glossier invisible shield, good for every day.

For a combined sunscreen, try: Obagi Tinted Sunshield SPF50 or SkinCeuticals Ultra Facial UV Defense SPF50 Sunscreen Protection.

You might think you are wearing enough sunscreen because there is SPF in your moisturizer and/or make-up. But I'd recommend a separate sunscreen, even so. Even I struggle to use the half teaspoon of sunscreen to give the labelled protection for face only; that's at least twice the amount of moisturizer most people apply.

However, if you must, must, *must* have a 'dual action' product, find one that is well formulated so it's high in broad spectrum SPF, that covers both UVA and UVB rays. Try: Paula's Choice Resist Skin Restoring Moisturiser SPF50.

There are some tinted sunscreens that give cover that might be just enough, such as Epionce Daily Shield Lotion Tinted SPF50. The problem can be colour matching, plus they can feel a little thick and pasty. But this is definitely an improving area, as there are lots of new options coming out. One last thing: fake tan is not sunscreen. It only gives an SPF of 3!

Basic 2: A close runner-up - cleanser

I focus on this step before moisturizers and serums - because getting it right is critical. Cleanser is the second most important step in your routine and should be used morning AND night. It removes oil, dirt, make-up - but also your skin's own products of metabolism that can build up and damage the function of your skin barrier.

My cleanser rule is: keep it gentle, and here's why. The acid mantle is a thin acidic film on the skin's surface composed of amino acids, fatty acids, sebum and lactate from sweat. Along with the skin microbiome, the protective layer of good bacteria on the skin, the acid mantle is part of the delicate matrix that creates a healthy skin barrier. Its main job is to protect from harmful bacteria and other microorganisms. Think of it as an essential shield - the invisible face mask you didn't know you were wearing.

Anything that skews the normal acidic pH of skin, which is between 4 and 6, can disrupt its ability to function optimally. And the biggest culprit is often cleanser.

Soap is alkaline (pH >7) and the surfactants in 'stronger' foaming cleansers disrupt the acid mantle too, dropping your skin's natural defences. The result is more bacteria. And that's the last thing acne sufferers who've turned to 'stronger' cleansers need!

Soaps and strong cleansers contain molecules called surfactants that bind to oil so that it can be washed away. But they also bind to your skin's essential components, such as proteins, lipids and a protective substance called natural moisturizing factor (NMF), stripping them away. And when some of these molecules are left behind, they penetrate the lipid matrix of your epidermis and cause prolonged irritation. These too-harsh cleansers also often contain extra ingredients to keep them in bar form or to foam. Your skin is a delicate balancing act - and these cleansers don't help!

How do you know this is happening to you? Ask yourself, how does my skin feel 20 seconds after cleansing?

Tight? This can be an indication that (a) your cleanser is too harsh; (b) your skin is irritated or dehydrated and has absorbed too much water during cleansing - which then evaporates fast, causing that very dry feeling.

The solution? Ban bar soaps and foaming cleansers. Castile soaps and even 'natural' soaps are too harsh. The same goes for the most common surfactant, sodium lauryl sulphate, found in most cleansers and also in house cleaners, shampoo and washing-up liquid. On labels, other too-harsh cleansers appear as sodium xx-ate - e.g. laurate/tallowate/cocoate.

Instead look for cleansers containing:

1. Milder surfactants. A mix is always better because then each ingredient will be less concentrated. Good ones are: SLES (sodium laureate sulphate); glucosides; xx-sarcosinate; xx-succinate; coconut-based amphoteric surfactants, 'cocoampho'.
2. Moisturizing ingredients, e.g. stearic acid, plant oils or humectants (e.g. glycerin, sorbitol). A good product to try is: La Roche Posay Toleraine dermo-cleanser.

What are the other rules for cleansing gently?

- NO to scrubs. They might feel as if they're giving a deeper clean, but very few skin types can really handle or benefit from these physical exfoliants, as they can cause abrasive damage and microtears. I prefer the chemical exfoliants, which can be both gentler *and* so much more effective.
- PROBABLY NO to facial brushes. These are just too irritating for most skin types. However, if you must use them, soft heads only, a maximum of 2-3 times per week, and CLEAN those heads regularly.
- NO to wipes. Not only are they not biodegradable, they leave a residue on your skin, so it's not properly cleansed.
- NO to hot water. It makes your (gentle) surfactants penetrate deeper and so can cause irritation. Yes to warm water.
- PERHAPS to massage techniques. These are hugely popular at the moment, and in general I am a fan. But be careful of vigorous techniques, as they can result in excessive tugging, especially around the eyes, and this can damage elastin fibres. There's more on massage in Chapter 6.

- YES to using a muslin or flannel. These are good if you really can't give up on that deep-clean feeling. But they're only really required at night to remove make-up and sunscreen. If you do use one twice a day, be gentle. In fact, be gentle full stop, as used with too much enthusiasm they can be as harsh as a brush or scrub. If your skin becomes at all sensitive, go back to using your fingertips temporarily.
- YES to alternating your usual cleanser with a stronger 'targeted' cleanser, for example one that includes mild acid exfoliants. But if you use these, don't use them twice a day, or even every day. Pay attention! A good one is: Neostrata Skin Active Exfoliating cleanser. For oily skin, try cleansers containing salicylic acid like Epionce Lytic Cleanser.

HOW TO REMOVE YOUR MAKE-UP

This may be a revelation to you, but you don't need make-up remover! It's an option, not a requirement. You only really need eye make-up remover.

So how to make sure you've taken all your make-up off and your skin feels really clean? Because I mostly recommend gentle cleansers, you can do this by double-cleansing, which is exactly what it sounds like: cleansing then cleansing again. Or by using a face cloth. This is a good way to make sure you've removed all your sunscreen, too. But only do this in the evening.

A balm or oil cleanser - such as Votary Oil Cleanser - may well remove all your make-up with a single cleanse using a cloth. If you are using vitamin A or other add-on ingredients (see page 141) you should then double-cleanse with a mild non-oil-based cleanser to remove surface residue before applying.

Or you can use a micellar water as your first cleanse, then follow up with your usual cleanser. Micellar waters are watery products that contain mild surfactants. Do always rinse or cleanse again after using them. Try: Bioderma Sensibio (*Crealine) H2O Make Up Removing Micelle Solution.

Which type of cleanser will suit you?

It may take some trial and error to find the one that works best. These are the ones I recommend:

- Milks and lotions or cold creams. Good for drier skin. My go-to in this category is Epionce Milky Lotion Cleanser - I give it to clients with redness and rosacea and when prepping them for laser for these treatments. In order for skin to feel really clean, you may need to double-cleanse or (gently) use your muslin or a face cloth.
- Basic foaming or gel cleanser. This is probably not the type to try if your skin is very dry, though CeraVe Foaming Facial Cleanser contains ceramides for moisture. They lather up once on your face.
- Self-foaming. A special pump means there's no need to lather up manually. These usually contain only mild surfactants; foaming is not an accurate measure of the strength of the surfactant!
- Oils and balms. Good for drier skin, best used with a cloth, and it can be lovely to leave some oil on your skin on nights when you are not using potent actives like vitamin A.
- Exfoliating cleansers. I am a fan. This is more of a treatment than a cleanse - so only use if your skin can handle it and only 2-3 times per week at most. (Oily skins may, however, tolerate and indeed benefit from more frequent use.) I often recommend Epionce Lytic Cleanser, which uses salicylic acid.

Basic 3: Vitamin A

This is the product that's worth investing in. You might have heard it called retinoids or retinol, and you'll definitely have heard the noise about how wonderful it is. So, what's all the fuss?

Vitamin A occurs naturally in our skin. The retinoids in skincare are a family of compounds derived from vitamin A. These include retinol, tretinoin (Retin-A is a brand name) and adapalene. Applying vitamin A gives your skin what I call a 'grown-up glow'. It's the gold standard for addressing all signs of skin ageing, effectively treating and preventing sun damage. It benefits every component of your epidermis and dermis, even down to the blood supply.

As vitamin A was originally used as a treatment for teenage acne, there's a wealth of clinical data on its impact. It was because of the research into acne that its other benefits were discovered, such as the fact that it has a direct impact on the cells of your dermis, stimulating them to produce new collagen. This is unlike all other skincare ingredients, which work indirectly and more superficially.

Vitamin A has been shown to act by influencing the expression of over 1,000 genes. It binds to DNA - via retinoid specific receptors - then turns on gene expression, directly triggering the production of new proteins, such as collagen and elastin, as well as blocking their breakdown.

Vitamin A basically does it all:

- Reduces fine lines and wrinkles
- Improves pore clarity and size
- Helps prevent spots
- Improves pigmentation
- Boosts collagen production

- Prevents the breakdown of collagen
- Acts as an antioxidant

So why isn't everyone using it already? As you can tell, vitamin A is my favourite skin changer. But I know you might be wary of using retinoids, as a lot of people are. If you're not already a convert, you might have tried them, then stopped, because you didn't like your skin's reaction to them, or because you didn't see a change. I'm going to explain that with the right formulation, and used the right way, most people can use Vitamin A.

How to start vitamin A

The process of starting a retinoid is called retinization. And it is ALWAYS a process, even for the hardiest of skins. About 4 or 5 days after you start using it, irritation will happen. Vitamin A is such a potent ingredient that, until your skin becomes used to it, it disrupts the barrier.

If you decide to go full on with a prescription-strength vitamin A, because you know you and your lifestyle can take it, and you are confident that you know what you are doing, it will take around 3 weeks to coax your skin into liking this. With a less strong product, the irritation may only last for a few days. But it's worth going through the retinization process: once your skin can tolerate vitamin A, the benefits are enormous.

Start slowly and build up

I see so many people who become blasé because their skin is fine on day 3, so they up their dose and frequency and then end up as a yo-yo user, having 4 days on, then 4 days off to recover.

Instead, use my 3-2-1-GO method (see page 133). Use it once a day (at night unless the product specifically states otherwise), every 3 days for 2 weeks, then every other day for 2 weeks. The eventual aim is to apply it every night, but there is no rush. Remember, this is an investment.

Start small and work up

A pea-size amount is plenty to begin with, working up to a 2cm stripe. I find it easier to be more precise with creams over pipettes. Again, it's all about being consistent. It's much better to start with the tiniest amount but use it regularly, then build up.

If you are going slowly and still experiencing too much irritation, here are a few tricks on how to manage it:

Pre-moisturize

Use moisturizer 5 minutes BEFORE applying the vitamin A, to buffer and dilute it. Then 5 minutes later, moisturize again. Use a moisturizer containing ceramides, niacinamide, or one that's richer than you would normally use for this retinization period, but aim to reduce that over the following weeks.

Go lightly on sensitive areas

You can either apply less or avoid these areas, such as around your eyes and mouth. Or you can apply a barrier first, such as lip balm or eye cream, 5 minutes before applying your vitamin A.

Massage it in

Apply to dry skin. Rub it in rather than leaving it to absorb.

Switch to an 'encapsulated' retinol

If this is on the label, it means it's formulated for slow release. These can sometimes ease side-effects. Try: Skinceuticals 0.3% Retinol.

How vitamin A is misunderstood

These are some of the most common questions and misunderstandings about vitamin A that I hear in the clinic.

'My skin doesn't do vit A.' / 'I'm allergic to retinoids.'

I hear this at least once a week. But the fact is, almost everybody will benefit from introducing a retinoid. Yes, you may experience side-effects when you first try them, and yes, your skin may perhaps become red, dry or flaky, but your skin *can* tolerate them.

If you have acne, rosacea or super-sensitive skin, you may struggle more than most to coax your skin into retinoid tolerance. And although it has been used for decades to treat adolescent acne, adult acne and indeed adult skin do often need to be handled more delicately. That's because underlying adult acne and/or rosacea, which often present together, there is usually inflammation, both of skin and at a deeper systemic level. This is different from adolescent acne, which is more about incessant pustule formation. So your threshold to irritation is already lower, and your skin is more likely to be reactive and also to take much longer to calm and repair. As an adult your higher level of stress and your slowed repair mechanisms also mean you need to go more carefully and slowly with introducing vitamin A. If you'd like more guidance and hand-holding, consult a doctor. You may just benefit from amazing results.

'I stopped because it's summer.'

The myth is that you can't use retinoids because they make your skin sensitive to the sun. This myth is a result of three things: it's recommended you don't use vitamin A in the sun, vitamin A can cause sensitivity when you first use it, and you're usually advised to apply vitamin A at night.

In reality, vitamin A doesn't make skin any more sensitive after the retinization period. The reason you're advised to use retinoids at night is because UV breaks down vitamin A, not because your skin is more at risk from UV when the product is on it. That's why you'll see your vitamin A comes in opaque packaging - to protect the product.

Research shows that vitamin A products do remain stable and effective under a sunscreen - as long as you use enough and reapply as necessary.

I do often advise my clients that summer is not the best time to start vitamin A, although it's fine to carry on using it. That's because you will always see a level of irritation (see retinization, page 124) in the first 6 weeks, and even if all the visible irritation stops quickly, your skin will be more sensitive.

Newer formulations that are more stable, such as those found in The Ordinary products are more stable in sunlight, and so can be used in the morning. Look for: 'Granactive retinoids' or 'novel retinoid' or 'hydroxypinacolone retinoate'.

However, if you plan to get a bit of a tan in the summer, maybe vitamin A is not for you. But if you are serious about skin, and if you want to use the gold standard product for your *# bestskinever* - now, or in 20 to 30/40 years - NO sun and NO tan (fake is OK!). Use a hat, glasses, and sit in the shade whenever possible. And obviously use sunscreen - reapplied every 2 hours if out in the sun, as sunlight breaks down the protective ingredients.

'I haven't peeled. It's not working.'
Vitamin A exfoliates differently to an acid exfoliant or scrub. It stimulates barrier cells to reproduce at the deeper layers and so speeds up turnover of dead cells at the surface. Flaking does not equal exfoliation. You do not need to flake and peel to reveal a smoother, renewed skin. Less or non-irritating cosmetic vitamin A products are still absolutely worth using!

'I've read that I shouldn't combine vitamin A products with acid exfoliants or vitamin C.'
Nooooo! These are skincare rumours that have sprung from a misunderstanding or misinterpretation of the research. They're rooted in a 20-year-old study that looked at how acidity impacts the way skin breaks down naturally occurring vitamin A. In fact, lowering

the pH of skin - making it more acidic - does not influence the action of vitamin A.

When you're starting out on vitamin A, I usually stop all other actives temporarily. But eventually, you can use them. This often gets you better results, for example when treating pigmentation. I'll usually rotate the two: exfoliant one night, vitamin A the next. And in the winter months, if skin is more sensitive, you can follow this with a rest night, too.

Finally, vitamin C actually helps retinoids work better because it breaks down the free radicals that can destabilize vitamin A.

Which vitamin A is right for you?

It's important to get both the concentration and the formulation right. These are some general guidelines:

For a little more brightness, better pore clarity, or if you're under 35

OTC (over the counter) formulations really do work for this, and are a great place to start. Try: GOW Granactive Retinoid 5% - which contains hydroxypinacolone retinoate.

For 35 plus

From your mid-30s, you could use either an over the counter or prescription product. However, most people won't see real benefits from a prescription product until they're 40 or older. Apply it nightly for 6 months. Then go down to using it 2 or 3 times per week, all year round. (Some people find that using vitamin A for 6 months then taking 6 months off works better with their lifestyle.)

To address acne, pigmentation, acne scarring and/or sun damage

Use a prescription strength product. Be prepared to stay out of the sun and take a few weeks downtime when your skin might not look its best.

Over the counter vs. prescription (Rx) strength: A simple guide

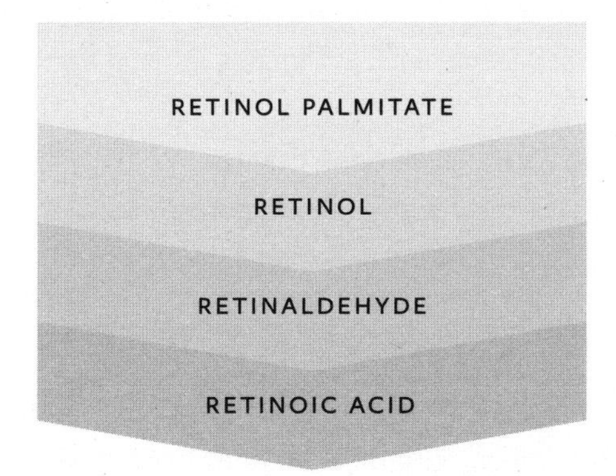

First, the strongest form of vitamin A is retinoic acid. This is found in prescription products only. When you apply this to your skin, it will bind directly to retinoid receptors and start the cascade of mechanisms that correct and prevent sun damage.

The other forms, available OTC, are 'storage' forms of vitamin A. That means they need to go through a step-by-step conversion process in your skin before starting those mechanisms. Each step required will reduce the potency of what you have applied tenfold.

A guide to over the counter forms of vitamin A

- Retinol palmitate. I tend not to use this. It has to go through 3 conversion steps to become active, so it has a pretty weak effect.
- A genuine 0.5–1% retinol can actually be as effective as a prescription product, it just takes longer. But a word of caution – it's almost impossible to know exactly what concentration you are actually getting. Ingredient labels are hard to decipher, as well as being misleading and notoriously inaccurate in this category. The possible variation in the actual concentration is enormous, from 0.01% to 1%. One worth trying is: Retriderm Max (1%).

- Retinaldehyde. 0.05%–0.1%. This is a good choice, 10 times stronger than retinol, and with good antibacterial properties, which is useful for acne. Try: Medik8, Crystal Retinal.

The following two forms have been created by manufacturers to act like retinoic acid and their formulas are extremely similar, but the difference is that they do not need a prescription.

- Granactive retinoid 'hydroxypinacolone retinoate'. This is the new kid on the block; it's early days but it looks to be a very interesting ingredient. A cosmetic ester of retinoic acid, it's more stable and less irritating and is able to bind to and directly activate the retinoid receptors, so no need for any conversion steps in the skin. Try: Votary Intense Night Oil, Sunday Riley Luna.
- Retinyl retinoate. This is an interesting combination product with both retinoic acid, which has direct impact and is very effective, and retinol, which is slow-release and better tolerated. Try: Medik8 r-Retinoate serum.

A guide to prescription-only forms of vitamin A

These are all versions of retinoic acid. If you have acne, you will be able to get a prescription from your GP. Otherwise, you'll need one from your dermatologist, private GP or skin clinic. You can do this online: Dermatica.co.uk is a service where your uploaded photos and questionnaire are reviewed remotely by a consultant dermatologist.

- Tretinoin (Brand names: Retin-A, Kettrel). Available in 3 concentrations: 0.025%, 0.05% and 0.1%. This is the gold standard for the repair of photo damage as a result of exposure to the sun.
- Adapalene (Brand name: Differin. This is available OTC in the US). Good for acne and pigmentation and typically causes much less irritation.

- Isotretinoin, which you take orally or apply in gel form. When combined with antibiotics for acne or rosacea, it's called Isotrexin.
- Tazarotene. This isn't a retinoic acid, but it's similar. It can be slightly more irritating, but it's very effective. As well as photo ageing, it treats acne and psoriasis.

Do not use vitamin A while pregnant or breastfeeding. It has been associated with foetal abnormalities when taken orally at prescription strength.

Basic 4: The glow giver - exfoliants

Exfoliants give a brilliant quick-ish cosmetic fix by removing dead skin cells from the surface. Well exfoliated skin looks bright and supple. But, as I'll explain, exfoliants have great functional benefits too.

My preferred option is a chemical exfoliator. These are acids that chemically dissolve the bonds, allowing the dead cells to come away more easily as you are washing your face. Despite sounding harsh, they can be pretty gentle. And there really is a chemical exfoliator for every skin type. Many of them don't sting at all, or cause any redness or visible peeling.

Some people use physical exfoliants, also called mechanical or abrasive, or a scrub. These physically break the bonds between the dead cells at the surface. As I've said, I don't like them. Very few skin types can actually handle them and even then, they're limited in how effective they can be.

So what are the functional benefits? Ageing causes the natural turnover process of your epidermis to slow down. In your teens the entire process - new cells forming in the basal layer, working their way up to the outer layer, flattening, dying and being shed - takes around

2 weeks. But by the time you are in your 40s this process can take 4 weeks or longer. The result: a build-up of dead cells on the surface. You'll notice the following signs of this build-up:

- Your skin feels rough.
- Your skin appears dull. That's because while the smooth surface of fresh cells revealed by exfoliation will reflect light, the uneven surface of dead cells will scatter it.
- You suffer from breakouts, as your pores become clogged by oils that soak up the dead cells.
- Your skin looks patchy and pigmented because melanocytes become oversensitive.
- Your products don't work as well because the dead cells block the active ingredients. Correct exfoliation allows products to penetrate better and so be more effective.

Consistent use of exfoliants brings improved hydration, as a better-functioning barrier layer leads to an increased ability to hold water. Some acid exfoliants, such as PHAs, are also humectants, which means they draw moisture into the skin. As skin becomes calmer and better hydrated, it leads to a direct improvement of the function of the deeper layers too, including enzymes and fibroblasts.

Which acid exfoliants are best for you?

I often recommend products that combine more than one acid, as they do all have slightly different effects:

- AHAs: Glycolic, lactic or mandelic acids. These are water-soluble. Glycolic is a stronger exfoliator, but lactic acid also binds water so it hydrates too. In fact lactic acid is a favourite of mine because it's a component of one of your skin's natural humectants, natural moisturizing factor (NMF). These are good for adding glow to all skin types.
- BHAs: Salicylic acid. It's oil soluble so it gets deeper into pores, and is great for congestion and spots. It's also

anti-inflammatory and antibacterial, so it's great for oily skin, as well as for acne and acne rosacea.
- PHAs: Gluconolactone. These are made up from larger molecules, and have slower absorption. They're hydrating and are great for more sensitive skin.

There are more organic alternatives to the acids I've mentioned above, such as the enzymes in pomegranate and pumpkin, but, honestly, they're not as effective. Having said this, if you prefer natural, they are a good place to start.

When a client has inflamed or hypersensitive skin, there may be priorities higher up the list such as retinoids. But most skins can usually take a BHA acid.

If you're still wary of chemical exfoliants, start slow and build up, using the 3-2-1-go method below.

3-2-1-GO METHOD

Use the product every 3 days for 2 weeks.
Then every other day for 2 weeks.
Finally you can use it every day. 3-2-1-go!

Basic 5: Defence and repair - antioxidant serum

When it comes to antioxidants, vitamin C really is the powerhouse. There is lots of evidence to show that it boosts your natural antioxidant system, fighting free radical damage, but also decreases the risk of sunburn by improving the effectiveness of sunscreens as well as protecting the skin's support structures.

Want more reasons to use it? It strengthens the skin barrier and stimulates new collagen synthesis. It improves pigmentation by blocking excess melanin production. It's anti-inflammatory, so it's good for skins that tend to acne and rosacea.

There are lots of different formulations of vitamin C. Because it oxidizes - goes off - when it's hit by light or air, it usually comes in dark packaging and small vials, or as a powder you mix up when needed. There can be some confusion over which type to use - mostly down to marketing hype - but there is really not much difference between them. Look for L-Ascorbic acid in the ingredients - the most potent form - starting at 10% and working up to 20%. Ascorbyl glucoside and magnesium ascorbyl phosphate (MAP) are also effective ingredients to look out for.

Using vitamin C is GOOD in pregnancy and very well tolerated. Use it once daily in the morning to support the function of your sunscreen, especially during the summer months, and if pigmentation is an issue. But you can use it in the afternoon for its repair benefits, too.

Try: Obagi Pro-C 10-20%. As I say, you should start at 10% and work up, though 15% is plenty enough for most skins. Balance Me Vitamin C Repair Serum is gentle and includes hyaluronic acid for hydration. Julia T. Hunter MD Vitamin C Plus is a powder that can be mixed in your palm with a few drops of water - great for those who don't get on with an oil-based serum.

What about moisturizer?

This is controversial: moisturizer doesn't make it to being a basic. Because not everybody needs a moisturizer every day and certainly not twice a day.

You might be thinking: but I can't do without mine. But moisturizers are over-hyped, and over-priced. Certainly a large percentage of my clients become less and less reliant on their moisturizer as their skin improves, and does the job it is designed to do - act as a shield that stops water from escaping.

Yes, your environment, for example pollution and changes in humidity, and your hormones, especially the menopause, can take a toll. So there will be times when your moisturizer will absolutely be essential. But the important, exciting ingredients - the ones that replenish and repair - are either (a) missing or not very active in many expensive moisturizers, and (b) often best found in a more concentrated serum.

So, shift your focus. Many clients spend their skincare budget on the fanciest moisturizer at the expense of other products. But if you are looking to invest in one, you don't need to get overwhelmed. The most important decision is texture - cream for dry skin, lotion for oily skin and so on (see page 136). Then, only apply it when and where it's needed.

What kind of moisturizer do you need?

All moisturizers have the same goal: to increase the water content of the stratum corneum. But they don't just do this by 'moisturizing'. They're usually a combination of ingredients with the three actions below. Most skins will benefit from having a little of each.

1. Preventing moisture evaporation from the skin using 'occlusive' ingredients. Usually oily, these coat the skin so water can't escape. Examples are: shea butter, lanolin, argan oil.

2. Strengthening of the skin barrier. You do this by using lipids that are naturally present in the skin, such as fatty acids, ceramides and cholesterol. I probably tell 90% of my clients that they need a ceramide-based moisturizer to support their barrier. You also do this with lighter-textured oils, called 'emollients', which means they soften and smooth the skin by

filling in the spaces between skin cells. Examples are: squalene and jojoba.

3. Increasing the ability of the skin to hold on to water, which you do with 'humectant' ingredients. Examples are: hyaluronic acid, urea (both natural components of the skin barrier), glycerin, alpha-hydroxy acids, honey.

If you have normal to dry skin and a light moisturizer is leaving your skin tight, before you switch to a rich cream, try adding a couple of drops of oil to it.

If you have very dry or sensitized, dehydrated skin, apply a humectant serum, for example hyaluronic acid, to damp skin, then an occlusive immediately afterwards. This will prevent any water drawn from the deeper layers of the epidermis from escaping.

If you have oily or acne-prone skin, you will still need moisturizing ingredients - even more so if you are using potent actives to address breakouts. Otherwise you are depriving your skin of key anti-ageing and barrier-strengthening ingredients. Try: Hydratime Plus. Occlusives are not great for oily skin, with the exception of silicones, which create a mesh over the skin rather than complete occlusion. All skin types should avoid comedogenic (pore-blocking) emollients such as coconut oil. Non-comedogenic ones include squalane and jojoba/ safflower oil. Try: Votary Super Seed Facial Oil.

Rule 2: Do no harm: why is your skin sensitive?

When clients tell me they have sensitive skin, they often assume it's down to their skin type or an allergy to a skincare ingredient. In fact, sensitivity is much more complex than that - and it's likely that by understanding the different factors you can transform your skin.

It's true that some people's skin is more reactive to certain products, especially to fragrances. But genuine ingredient allergies are NOT common at all. If you have had what you think is an 'allergic reaction' to a product, it's more likely because of its formulation, using alcohol and/or fragrance.

Fragrances, both synthetic and natural, are the most common cause of sensitizing skin and allergic reactions. There are 26 recognized fragrance allergens listed in the 'EU Cosmetic Regulation'. And these include natural products, such as the essential oils of rose, lemongrass, Ceylon cinnamon, apple, apricot, cassis, blackberry, blueberry, orange, passion fruit and peach. If you think your product is to blame, I'd advise cutting it out - I'll explain how to do this in the intervention programme on page 152.

But it's not usually these ingredients that explain 95% of the cases of sensitivity I see in the clinic. They are in fact due to the following three reasons - which will also be helped by the intervention programme.

Overload

The majority of 'sensitivity' cases I see in the clinic are simply down to clients using too many active products at once. It's not that skin is innately sensitized, it's that skin has become sensitized. Throw in regular peels and/or medical facials, or regular massage with fragranced oils or overly stimulating devices, and your skin will behave as hypersensitive and reactive. Even if you have been using the same products for ages with no adverse results, there may be a tipping point into sensitivity. It's not the product per se that's the cause, but that your skin's reserves are maxed out.

Systemic inflammation

I've written about inflammation in depth in Chapter 1. But to reiterate: our lifestyles mean inflammation is now the natural state of most of our bodies, most of the time. And when sensitive skin presents, it's often lurking in the background, a key underlying cause. You can tackle it by making some of the lifestyle changes suggested in Chapter 3.

You're using the wrong products for your skin type and/or concern

Remember, you are an individual and the products you use and the regime you follow will be personal to *you*. Skincare decisions need to take into account so many factors, from genetics and lifestyle, to budget and more. Try to remember this when you are enjoying content from skinfluencers and brand ambassadors. The skincare that's right for them may not be right for you.

I see a lot of people who avoid moisturizer because they have oily skin. That's skin that is prone to blackheads and spots, but also skin that looks shiny in pictures; you have large pores and your make-up slides off during the day. If this is you, do use moisturizer but choose a liquid gel formula.

I also see people who choose too-thick moisturizers, especially night creams. Normal to oily skin should choose gels, liquids and the thinner-textured lotions.

If you have blackheads and bumps, you may assume you have combination skin and hold back on moisturizer too. But congestion can happen in dry skin, even if your skin looks matte and make-up settles in fine lines. Do keep using moisturizer and you will also benefit from an acid exfoliant (see page 131).

If you have very dry skin, you do need rich creams. But normal to dry skin will find this too heavy, and will do better with a lotion or lighter cream. Or consider a reset programme (see page 144).

Making the switch to active skincare

Now we're going to start to build on your skincare routine. As I've said, active, targeted ingredients and concentrated formulations are the way to both cosmetic and functional improvements. They are ONLY to be started on skin that's been prepped (see the reset and Intervention programmes on pages 143–56).

Which products are really active?

My philosophy is: good ingredients, good formulations and good evidence are far more important than packaging or brands. I choose the brands I use in the clinic because they have a higher concentration of actives, they are well formulated and they have more clinical trials and data than other brands.

That said, there is far less difference between clinic, medical-grade or cosmeceutical (having more than just a cosmetic impact) products and over the counter brands than there was just a few years ago. Now, so many products that would have been termed 'medical-grade' 5 years ago, such as acid exfoliants and some antioxidant serums, are available OTC.

In fact, pretty much all products that you'd call cosmeceutical, medical-grade or clinical are available OTC or online now. If they're not it is usually a brand decision rather than down to their formulation. Prescription-only products are, of course, more potent and the exception to this.

These are the brands of skincare that I use every day in the clinic: Epionce; Obagi Nu-Derm, Neostrata, Julia T. Hunter MD, ZO Skin health, Medik8 and Tebiskin. I'll often use them in combination with the professional strength treatments and peels of the same brands. Other fantastic brands are: Skinceuticals, iS Clinical and Skinbetter Science. You can buy most of them online; try getharley.com, who connect you with aesthetic professionals who create personalized online skincare plans.

That's not to say that my clients do not get good results from other non-clinic brands, a few of which I'll also mention throughout the chapter.

When I say a product is well formulated, it means that what is on the label is what goes into your skin. Just because a product is branded 'medical' does not guarantee this.

Some products lose effectiveness even while on the shelf. For example, vitamin C is known to be super-unstable, as it oxidizes as soon as you open the bottle. But one vitamin C product I use, Tebiskin SOD-C , has over 85% proven efficacy, even 3 weeks after opening the bottle. This is unlike many vitamin C products sold over the counter.

It also means they have effective delivery of the active ingredients. Remember, most ingredients are simply too large to be absorbed into the skin. But good formulations are those where ingredients have been shown to get into the skin.

My message is: it's time to move beyond luxury or designer brands such as La Prairie, Sisley, Crème de la Mer. There is nothing wrong with the old school, such as Clarins, Decléor, Estée Lauder, but there are so many exciting new ranges that use great technology, and have a great price point. The Ordinary, GOW, Beauty Pie, The Inkey List: these are true disruptors with effective products starting from under £10. Some products are really worth investing in, too: Oskia, Murad, Ren and DDG are among my favourite brands available over the counter.

And if you're not prepared to wave goodbye to the indulgence and ritual of those beautifully packaged, scented elixirs, then don't! There is nothing wrong with that - I like them too - but focus on ingredients over brands.

So this is where to spend your money! But only once you've got your basics. To address more severe skin issues such as signs of ageing and sun damage, skin texture, wrinkling and uneven tone, or problem skin, you'll need to top up your BASICS with some TARGETED skincare.

My Top 5 targeted add-ons

Once you've got your basics right, these are the super-charging ingredients I rate.

Hyaluronic acid (HA)

Your skin produces this, but levels go down with age. The skincare version comes as a serum or spray, for example Teoxane RHA Serum. It's a good humectant, best used in combination with an occlusive to stop moisture drawn from the skin from escaping. The molecules are too large to be absorbed, so it sits on the surface of the skin. The most effective way to use it is Profhilo, a skin booster where tiny amounts are injected all over the skin, which gives a lovely plumping effect as well as a glow. This version is not strictly skincare, but it's one that's only getting more popular.

Azelaic acid

This occurs naturally in the skin and is produced by your skin's microbiome. It's also found in wheat and barley. It's anti-inflammatory, as it actually dials down an over-sensitized immune system in rosacea; anti-bacterial; anti-comedonal and an antioxidant. It's available OTC as well as prescription strength. It also blocks melanin formation so is great for treating pigmentation. Try: Paula's Choice 10% Azelaic Acid Booster (15% and 20% require a prescription).

Niacinamide (vitamin B3)

This works for every sign of skin ageing.

In dry, dull skin, it boosts production of ceramides in the skin barrier, so it helps with hydration.

For redness, it's anti-inflammatory, so it's great for angry, sensitive skin including acne and rosacea.

For pigmentation, it blocks melanin transfer from where it's produced to where you see it. It works well with azelaic acid or hydroquinone because it blocks at a different stage of the pigment formation pathway.

For wrinkles and sagging, it improves energy production in your skin, so boosting repair and regeneration, new collagen, elastin and your skin's own HA production.

Plus, it's very well tolerated and can be used in pregnancy and breastfeeding. Try: ELTA MD PM Therapy, a great lightweight moisturizer (also in their sunscreen CLEAR) or Glossier Super Pure.

Bakuchiol

This is an exciting new plant-derived ingredient. It behaves like a retinoid, but without the irritation and instability. It's anti-inflammatory, anti-bacterial and a powerful antioxidant. It also boosts collagen, elastin and HA levels in the dermis by stimulating production and blocking breakdown. Finally, it's good for pigment – blocking two key stages of the melanin production process. Plus, it can be used day and night, as it's not broken down by UV rays like vitamin A is. Try: Medik8 Bakuchiol Peptides.

Peptides

These are 'cell-communicating' ingredients, skin messengers that help to repair and regenerate on multiple levels. They are definitely not the miracle ingredients they've been cracked up to be, but they are worth considering if you have money to spend on an extra serum. Try: Neostrata Tri Therapy Lifting Serum.

The Programmes

I've devised some specialized programmes to suit the needs of different skin. These broadly follow what I'd do in the clinic based on the latest science. They do require some investment of time and money as well as staying power. But think of all the money you might have wasted on skincare that hasn't worked! In the clinic, I can add maintenance and regenerative treatments (see Chapters 6 and 7) too, but they work as stand-alone programmes.

Stage 1 of each programme is always about stripping back. That means using only cleanser, moisturizer and sunscreen for a period of weeks or months, depending on your skin. If you don't have a history of irritation and/or sensitized skin, it may be for just a week or two. If you do, it may be up to 6 weeks.

In Stage 2 you'll add an antioxidant, an acid exfoliant and/or a vitamin A.

Stage 3 is the add-on and maintenance stage, where you'll introduce targeted ingredients, always keeping an eye on your skin to see what's working.

There are two types of programme:

RESETS are to strengthen and boost skin. There are three versions: one for skin that's dehydrated and dull, one for mature skin where your concerns are wrinkles or sagging, and one for pigmentation. The one for dull skin will also suit you if you don't have a particular concern, but you just want your skin to look better.

INTERVENTIONS will calm sensitized skin that tends to redness or flushing. These are also for rosacea and acne, but these conditions may need a clinic visit and/or prescription, as well as lifestyle changes (see Chapter 3).

As you know, vitamin A is my hero product. But don't use it if you plan to conceive in the next year. It's not dangerous but it can take a year to achieve its full effect, so it may be a waste of time to start. Also, don't do this step if you're going on a sunny beach or ski holiday in the first 6 weeks of using it.

There are some essentials that will help you make sure you're getting the most out of your programme.

1. Detox your shelves of all the products you've tried that haven't worked so far. Don't worry: you may be able to add some back in. However, I'd recommend you bin harsh cleansers (see page 119).
2. Stick to the programme for the full time suggested. Remember, good skin takes time. There are no quick fixes.
3. Be consistent. For results, you'll need to stick to the same products too. No switching up!

I have also included the steps from these programmes in easy-to-follow tables at the back of the book (from page 266), to show you exactly what to do each day, a.m. and p.m.

THE RESET for dull and dehydrated skin

This is for you if: Your skin has lost its glow. Your usual products and facials just aren't having the same impact any more. You're tired of spending so much time and money following the advice of bloggers or sales staff. You find yourself wearing more and more make-up, which is starting to settle in early fine lines.

Stages 1 and 2 will take a minimum of 12 weeks, as you slowly introduce new products one at a time. This programme applies to over the counter vitamin A. If you are using a prescription product, follow your practitioner's instructions.

Stage 1: Strip back

WEEKS 1 AND 2: Cut down to 3 products only: cleanser, moisturizer, sunscreen. Often clients are using more than 6 products (scrub, mask, toner, serums and so on) and/or regularly changing brands. Your skin will thank you for keeping things minimal.

- Gentle cleanser, with very low dose acid exfoliants instead of harsh surfactants. Try: Skin Therapy by Julia T. Hunter MD Cleanser. This has very mild surfactants plus gluconolactone, a mild, hydrating PHA. Epionce Gentle Foaming Cleanser includes willow bark extract, which is a botanical source of salicylic acid, plus marshmallow extract and omega-3+ fatty acids, which soothe and boost hydration.
- Moisturizer. Choose one with strengthening and calming ingredients. Good ingredients to look for are ceramides, squalene, allantoin, the herb feverfew and oats. Try: Epionce Renewal Cream with avocado and flax oils for barrier strength plus antioxidants and anti-inflammatories. CeraVe Moisturising Cream for Dry to Very Dry Skin if dryness is your main issue.
- Sunscreen. This is the most important part of Stage 1: start wearing sunscreen every day. Find one you're happy with: I usually begin with as light a formulation as possible. Try: Elta MD Clear. If you prefer a tinted sunscreen to replace your foundation, try: Neostrata Sheer Physical Protection SPF50 or ZO Oclipse Sunscreen and Primer.

Stage 2: Treat

WEEKS 3 TO 12

This is the introduction of the 3 As: acid exfoliant, antioxidant serum, vitamin A. Be aware that during this stage, while your skin acclimatizes, you may have some mild irritation including temporarily dry, tight skin and occasional breakouts.

WEEKS 3 TO 5: Start using a leave-on acid exfoliant. Try: Epionce Lytic Tx or Beauty Pie Plantastic Micropeeling Drops. Use every evening. Moisturize 5 minutes after applying.
WEEKS 6 TO 8: Add an antioxidant serum. Try: Obagi Pro-C 15%. Use every morning.
WEEKS 9 TO 12: Add vitamin A (see page 128 for the one that's right for you), every 3 days, leaving 20 minutes before moisturizing. Rotate with your other products as per the table. Beauty Pie Super Retinol (+Vitamin C) Night Renewal Moisturizer is a gentle but effective non-prescription option.

If vitamin A isn't appropriate, step up your exfoliation. Try: Obagi Clenziderm 2% Salicylic Acid Toner, Skin Therapy by Julia T. Hunter MD Exfoliating Repair (lactic acid), or Epionce Lytic Cleanser (salicylic acid). Use twice per week.

Stage 3: Maintenance

WEEKS 13+

If your skin needs a hydration boost, add either niacinamide or hyaluronic acid on the days you're not using vitamin A. Try: Epionce Intense Defense Serum, Paula's Choice 10% Niacinamide Booster, Skin Therapy by Julia T. Hunter MD Wrinkle Filler (HA).

Another optional add-on is to start using an exfoliating cleanser twice a week.

THE RESET for mature skin

This is for you if: Your skin looks dull and lifeless, crêpey or you have wrinkles. Perhaps you've noticed you're reaching for richer and richer moisturizers but your skin is still looking lacklustre?

As you age and especially towards the menopause, skin tends to produce less sebum and so becomes drier as well as being less able to hold on to moisture, i.e. it becomes more dehydrated. The amount of damage in the dermis increases and there's a slowing down of the production of structural collagen and elastin. Skincare can do a lot: it can target fine lines and the loss of plumpness that's a very early sign of sagging, leaving skin looking brighter and with better tone and glow. What it can't do is treat deeper wrinkles or sagging due to volume loss, which do best with a clinic visit (see Chapter 7 onwards). Follow the lifestyle advice in Chapter 3 at the same time as this programme: glow comes from the inside.

Stage 1: Strip back

WEEKS 1 AND 2: Cut down to 3 key products.

- First things first: sunscreen. It is possible to find one that won't cause breakouts. Mature skins can often take the thicker formulas, which give more cosmetic cover. Try: Epionce Daily Shield Tinted spf50 or Obagi Matte Sunshield SPF50.
- Oil or balm cleanser. For these first 2 weeks, you'll leave the film of oil on your skin for moisture. Try: Votary Cleansing Oil or Clinique WTDA.
- Moisturizer. You may have been using expensive, luxury serums and moisturizers for years, and may not want to give them up because you like the way they make your skin look. But often, this effect is cosmetic, a glow, blur or sheen that comes from ingredients such as smoothing silicon or clever light diffusing particles. Tip: apply moisturizer to damp skin, to trap the surface moisture. Try: Epionce Intensive Nourishing Cream. This is our best seller. It's a rich moisturizer but also contains meadowfoam extract, a source of fatty acids that calm and strengthen. If you want something lighter, Epionce Renewal Lotion is packed with avocado and flax extracts that are anti-inflammatory and boost the skin barrier. Or CeraVe Moisturising Cream for Dry to Very Dry Skin.

Stage 2: Treat

WEEKS 3 TO 12

WEEKS 3 TO 5: Begin doing a second cleanse using a cloth to take off the oil, so you get maximum effect from your active ingredients. Introduce an exfoliant. Start by using it 2 days on, 1 day off, gradually building up to every night - but only when your skin can tolerate it. Try: Neostrata Skin Active Cellular Restoration, a great combined exfoliant and moisturizer, good for those who don't have very dry skin. Or instead try an acid toner, such as Biologique Recherche Lotion P50, a combination of acid exfoliants.

WEEKS 6 TO 8: Add antioxidant serum. Try: Neostrata Skin Active Antioxidant Defense Serum, which is a combination of 8 antioxidants.

WEEKS 9, 10: Add vitamin A. This is absolutely key to this programme. Use the 3-2-1-Go method (see page 124) and start by using it once every 3 days, following the table. In clinic, I'll often go straight to prescription strength. You can also try: Skin Therapy by Julia T. Hunter MD Vitamin A Plus, or Neostrata Skin Active Retinol + NAG Complex.

WEEKS 11, 12: Start using your vitamin A every other day, as per the table. Only use your acid exfoliant when your skin can tolerate it.

Stage 3: Add-ons

WEEKS 13+

You can move to using vitamin A every night for 6 months, after which you can cut down (see page 128 for more). Once your skin is happy with this, with no irritation, you can move to optional add-ons. You can add as many as you want, but one at a time, and use each one for 2 weeks before you add another.

- Hyaluronic acid for hydration. Try: Teoxane RHA Serum.
- Peptides will boost collagen. Try: Neostrata Tri-Therapy Lifting Serum, or Boots Protect and Perfect Serum no.7.
- Bakuchiol boosts collagen and elastin without the irritation that comes with vitamin A. Try: Medik8 Bakuchiol Peptides.
- Niacinamide. Try: Epionce Intense Defence Serum.

CASE STUDY

Anna, aged 57, came to see me feeling desperate about her appearance and asking for BTX and fillers. She told me she had spent thousands of pounds on beauty products. She'd bought and tried so many different brands, most of which were natural. She had shelves of oils and serums. She loved the ritual of using them – but she was sick of not seeing any change in her skin. In fact, quite the opposite: not only did she think her skin was looking older, but she had developed spots around her mouth, too.

The first thing I did was put her on the reset regime for mature skin, which starts with 3 products: a gentle cleanser, a light moisturizer and sunscreen. Having to go down to basics, she felt bereft of all her luxury oils, serums and creams. I told her that once her skin's barrier was restored, she'd no longer get breakouts and her skin would look glowier and plumper without a gloopy, heavy moisturizer – and eventually she'd be able to go back to some of her products.

Anna didn't want to try what she thought of as 'chemical' products – particularly sunscreen. But she agreed to using sunscreen after I explained its importance and she wanted results. Once she found one that was comfortable, she was fine about wearing it every day.

After 2 weeks, Anna began using an acid exfoliant with salicylic acid (Epionce Lytic Tx), which takes off the dead skin cells as you wash your skin, with no scrubbing, stinging or flaking. A week later, she said she noticed a glow. And a week after that, her spots started to improve too. On week 9, I started Anna on vitamin A (tretinoin 0.025%), which she's still using. Vitamin A takes time to work: recent research shows that you get a real difference in the dermis after using it for a year.

Six months into her programme, Anna's skin is plumper and more supple. In fact, she feels so much more confident in the way it looks that she has decided not to have fillers. She did have a little BTX in her frown lines and crows' feet, but much less than she would have had without the skincare reset.

THE RESET for pigmentation

This programme will only reduce the appearance of the pigmentation you have now. So it's important to establish the cause, in order to stop it happening for good. Is it down to hormones, for example melasma from being on the Pill or from pregnancy? There is often an element of systemic inflammation from stress involved in pigmentation too, and changing your lifestyle can help here (see Chapter 3). Or is it down to having breakouts? If that is the case, treat this issue before you start this reset (see the advice for acne, page 154). And remember: sun avoidance and sunscreen is key *for ever*, if you are serious about treating pigmentation.

This is usually a prescription regime: the gold standard treatment is prescription strength hydroquinone at 4%. If you don't want to use this, there are non-prescription options (see page 151).

Stage 1: Strip back

WEEKS 1 AND 2

Use the same recommendations as for the reset for dull and dehydrated skin (page 144). Simplifying your regime is a great idea, because over-stimulating skin is a trigger for pigmentation.

Stages 2 and 3: Treat

WEEKS 3 TO 12

A combination of vitamin C, acid exfoliant and vitamin A will help treat pigmentation and is what you'll continue to use once you've stopped the hydroquinone, for maintenance. (Do not use vitamin A and acid exfoliant together unless you are using hydroquinone, as it could possibly worsen pigment.)

I often prescribe the Obagi Nu-Derm system in the clinic, which includes all these elements. It can be an excellent reset programme for mature skin too. All products in the system are available separately too, although Obagi Nu-Derm Tretinoin and the hydroquinone 4% are only available on prescription.

For a non-prescription alternative to hydroquinone, the ingredients to look for are: azelaic acid, kojic acid, liquorice, tranexamic acid, niacinamide. Try: Epionce Melanolyte Tx with liquorice extract and Epionce Pigment Perfection Serum which contains anti-inflammatories and antioxidants.

WEEKS 3 TO 5: Add in acid exfoliant and prescription hydroquinone or non-prescription pigmentation serum, as per the table (see page 270). Take both actives to the hairline and as far as the orbit bone, not on to the neck.

WEEKS 6 TO 12: Add antioxidant serum and prescription vitamin A (tretinoin) as per the table (see page 272). Start with a pea-sized amount. (You may need to use them for more than 12 weeks to get the result you want.)

Stage 4: maintenance

WEEK 13+

Do not stop hydroquinone abruptly. It must be weaned off over 4 weeks to prevent rebound hyperpigmentation. From week 12 onwards, you can include add-ons for other skin concerns, but do it slowly as per the other programmes. See the table for details.

CASE STUDY

Liz, aged 38, told me she was going to a big school reunion in three months' time. And what she wanted was for her skin to look really stand-out by then. She had a little pigmentation but her skin was generally stable. She was busy at work and said she didn't have time to come in for lots of treatments.

I told her that vitamin A would give her the results she was looking for, but that her skin might become sensitized for a few weeks. She said, 'I don't care if I flake, just give me the chemicals!' I put her on the Obagi Nu-Derm home programme, which takes 12 weeks. Although it does need to be supervised at a clinic, it only requires visits at week 6 and 11, and then the rest can usually be done virtually. Liz did have some sensitization and peeling from the vitamin A in the first few weeks, but by the time her reunion happened, her skin was looking smoother, more even and much more glowy – even without make-up.

THE INTERVENTION for sensitized skin

This is for you if your skin often feels tight, and flushes easily. Or it has a rough or dry texture with occasional breakouts. Or it's red and angry. Or it's erratic, sometimes calm but unpredictable. Or it's increasingly sensitive to various products. Or you're wearing more and more make-up.

This programme is also what I would use to prepare a client for a course of laser treatment. When it comes to sensitized skin, it's a good idea to tackle the body's systemic inflammation too – for more on this, see Chapter 3.

I've also included versions for acne or acne rosacea below, but these conditions really do need to be treated in clinic. I usually combine prescription skincare with procedures such as peels (page 192) and lasers (page 209).

Stage 1: Strip back

WEEKS 1 TO 6

Avoid fragrances. That includes 'parfum' and essential oils. Also avoid scrubs and/or granules, acid cleansers, very hot water - no long hot showers.

- Gentle cleanser twice per day. Try: Epionce Milky Lotion Cleanser, Avène Extremely Gentle Cleansing Lotion.
- Moisturizer with barrier-strengthening ingredients and anti-inflammatories, e.g. ceramides, feverfew, chamomile, azelaic acid or niacinamide. Try: Epionce Renewal Soothing Cream, Avène Cicalfate+ Restorative Protective Cream, CeraVe Moisturising Lotion.
- Sunscreen. Try: Heliocre 360 Water Gel SPF50. I very rarely say this, but if your skin is flaring up, you may need to omit sunscreen for a few days. The number of chemicals in even the purest sunscreen can be too much. But stay out of the sun - when skin is inflamed, its threshold to UV damage is at its lowest.

Stage 2: Treat

WEEKS 7 TO 12

WEEKS 7 TO 9: Leave-on exfoliant - salicylic acid is often my first choice. Try: Epionce Lite Lytic Tx, which also contains azelaic acid - a great targeted add-on (see page 154).

WEEKS 10 TO 12: Vitamin C serum. Try: Skin Therapy by Julia T. Hunter MD Vitamin C Plus. You mix this powder with drops of water or her serum in your palm before applying. If this is still too sensitizing, add a couple of drops of Skin Therapy by Julia T. Hunter MD Emu Oil to the mix. Magnesium ascorbyl phosphate is a water soluble alternative that's usually less irritating.

Stage 3: Add-ons

FROM WEEK 13+

- Add targeted ingredients one at a time, waiting 2 weeks between them.
- Azelaic acid (usually prescription strength). Try: The Ordinary Azelaic Acid Suspension 10%.
- Niacinamide. Or try: Epionce Intense Defence Serum.

THE INTERVENTION for rosacea

Follow the plan for sensitized skin as above, but skip the acid exfoliant and vitamin C serum while skin is inflamed, sore or if you have any spots.

If there is no response to the reset within 6 to 12 weeks, it's worth going on to prescription products, which you'll get from your GP or a dermatologist. These may include azelaic acid, metronidazole and ivermectin. The clinic option at this point is laser treatments, but do not have these if your skin is very inflamed or you can see pustules.

THE INTERVENTION for adult acne

You've probably been told that acne is an oily skin condition, but so often the breakouts I see are caused by sensitized skin. Inflamed skin produces more sebum, and dead skin cells that have accumulated soak in this sebum and begin to clog pores. This allows acne bacteria to flourish. Drying out your skin, i.e. cleansing harshly, almost always worsens inflammation and results in your skin producing more sebum.

The intervention programme will suit you if your acne isn't too aggressive or at the early stages of a flare-up. Moderate to severe acne often requires prescription strength products. But I rarely go straight to antibiotics: there is so much that can be done before this - a nutritional approach, peels and laser facials - but it will require patience.

Hormones and/or stress are often at the root, so you need to look at your lifestyle too (see Chapter 3). The ideal is that you treat your skin from the outside while you address your lifestyle, then you're able to come off prescription skincare within 6 months. That said, acne is a condition that will need ongoing management.

Stage 1: Strip back

WEEKS 1 TO 6

- Even if you're tempted to use a harsh cleanser, don't! They will make things worse. Try: Dr Sam's Flawless Cleanser.
- Don't omit moisturizer even if it feels counter-intuitive. Try: Hydratime Plus or Neutrogena Hydro Boost Water Gel Moisturiser.
- At the same time, I'll often add a prescription cream. That might be Differin (contains adapalene, a retinoid), or Duac (contains benzoyl peroxide and an antibiotic).
- Sunscreen. This is especially important to allow you to move on to stages 2 and 3. Try: Elta MD Clear.

Stage 2: Treat

WEEK 7 TO 12, OR UP TO WEEK 24

For acne, this stage can last up to 6 months. Use prescription strength vitamin A according to your practitioner's instructions. This not only decreases sebum production but also helps exfoliation and repairs skin post-inflammation.

- Salicylic acid. This is anti-inflammatory as well as brilliant at improving turnover of pore lining cells, reducing the risk of clogging. You can use it morning or night but not at the same time as vitamin A, as this may make inflammation worse. Try: Epionce Lytic Sport if skin is inflamed, and Clenziderm Pore Therapy (2%) once it's calmer. If you need a treatment to apply directly to spots, try: Neostrata Targeted Clarifying Gel.

- Vitamin C antioxidant serum is good for skin repair but do use with caution and stop if any irritation. Also, most vitamin C serums are oil based, so try: Skin Therapy by Julia T. Hunter MD Vitamin C powder.

Stage 3: Maintenance

WEEKS 13+ (OR 25+)

For extra treatment when needed, try these add-ons:

- Benzoyl peroxide, for example acnecide (5%), destroys bacteria and helps exfoliate clogged pores.
- Clinisept is an antibacterial solution. Use it immediately after cleansing.
- Azelaic acid. This is anti-inflammatory, antibacterial and unclogs pores.
- Niacinamide is anti-inflammatory, reduces oil production and encourages ceramide production.

Extra skincare stages

People often ask me if they can keep using these products:

Toners

You may love the fresh feel of your skin after a toner. But toners should not be astringent or alcohol based to 'shrink pores', or 'dry oil'. That kind of toner is way too harsh. Instead, I like the kind of toner that rebalances your skin's pH after cleanser and preps it for the next skincare step. 'Essences' are an example of the new toner that preps, e.g. Exuviance Probiotic Lysate Anti-Pollution Essence (PHA (mild exfoliating acid) + hyaluronic acid). Or look for calming ingredients, e.g. Medik8 Daily Refresh Balancing Toner (glycerin, niacinamide and allantoin). If you don't have time for this step, I'd say it's one you can skip.

Eye creams

These are not complete hype. Ideally, your facial skincare will do the job. But the under-eye area has thinner skin and fewer oil glands, so if you are using a super light moisturizer, you may want to try them. The same is true if the eye area feels too sensitive for your active skincare - feel free to invest. Try: ZO Hydrafirm Eye Brightening Repair Crème, which includes ingredients to tackle pigment and puffiness, or Epionce Renewal Eye Cream for calming and hydrating.

Tips:

- Benefit to dark circles or puffiness will be minimal - and probably transient.
- Apply before moisturizer because you want the active ingredients to go straight on to the skin.

Neck creams

Again, you don't necessarily need a separate product here. You should include your neck in all your skincare routine, as well as your hands. They are often forgotten but benefit hugely from TLC. The neck is not an area where you should hold back on moisturizer: go rich! And if you are using particularly strong actives on your face (for example, tretinoin), be careful on your neck as it is more sensitive and less tolerant of downtime. You may want to buffer it with moisturizer first.

Living with a chronic skin condition can be truly confidence-crushing. It holds so many people back from living their fullest life. We have mentioned a few of these conditions before when talking about lifestyle medicine and how our diet, stress, sleep and pollution can affect our skin. But there is also help out there when it comes to active skincare. However, you will need to accept that self-prescribed home regimes are, often, not enough. If you suffer with persistent or recurrent acne, scarring, pigmentation, rosacea or psoriasis, speak to your GP about being referred to a dermatologist. Also, consider seeking help in an aesthetic clinic.

MIRACLE PRODUCTS OR MARKETING GIMMICKS?

Every week there seems to be a new must-have product that every skinfluencer and brand ambassador cannot live without. Here are a few from recent years and my thoughts on them:

- **Facial massage tools**
  These might be gua sha tools, jade rollers, rose quartz rollers. Fun! If they motivate you to spend time on massage and lymphatic drainage, to relax and unwind - go for it.

- **Sheet face masks**
  If you have the time and money and you enjoy the experience, by all means use these. But if you find yourself reaching for them regularly because you think your skin needs them, then you need to take a look at your daily skincare. There is nothing in these sheet masks that shouldn't already be covered in your routine. Masks are also questionable when it comes to their impact on the environment, so try to find one you know for sure is biodegradable.

- **Home LED Mask**
  I'm a fan of LED and the principle behind it is sound. I have two concerns. Using our strong clinic machine you need a minimum of 20 minutes, twice per week, for noticeable, visible improvements. Is the mask strong enough to make a real difference? And the second is, will you really keep doing it?

Rule 3: Pay attention - what are your skincare concerns?

Just as I would in the clinic, I would like you to evaluate your skin and think about the issues that bother you and what you would like to change. You might recognize yourself in some of the clients I have met over the years:

YOU ARE: The self-prescriber. Space NK loyalty card holder and beauty shopper extraordinaire.
I SUGGEST: The reset for dull and dehydrated skin (page 144). You are ready to transform with a shorter regime that works.

YOU ARE: The sceptic. You use water and Weleda Skin Food only.
I SUGGEST: Upgrade to active skincare (page 110). It's time to get serious.

YOU ARE: Someone who never leaves the house without make-up. You've tried everything - and you're allergic to it! Nothing works.
I SUGGEST: The intervention for sensitized skin (page 152). Plus lifestyle issues: in particular, let's take a look at your stress levels (see Chapter 3).

YOU ARE: Someone with an inflammatory skin condition such as acne or rosacea.
I SUGGEST: A combination. Try the intervention programme for acne (page 154). Then take a look at your diet, your stress levels and perhaps your hormone balance (see Chapter 3). In terms of a treatment programme, I'd suggest you kick off with a medical facial and LED (see Chapter 6), then move on to regenerative laser treatments for scarring, plus optimizing treatments for pigmentation/ dilated vessels (see Chapter 8) in the maintenance stage.

What's your skin status?

Use this questionnaire to monitor your skin before and during your new skincare regime. This will help you know what's working, and what you don't like. You might just be amazed at the progress you make. Remember Rule 3: Pay attention!

Fill in the following boxes, then score yourself for your skin status.

WHAT DO I LIKE ABOUT MY SKIN?	WHAT WOULD I LIKE TO IMPROVE?

What do you see?

Give yourself a score for each of these based on your *current* skin status, then add the total up at the end to work out what your result is.

1. Dull, dehydrated
   (0) Radiant
   (1) Not as bright, lacklustre
   (2) Tight, sallow, losing my glow
   (3) Sometimes flaky, feels rough
2. Redness
   (0) No redness
   (1) Some red dots, I use concealer around my nose
   (2) Red/sensitive cheeks
   (3) Sore, spots sometimes
3. Pigmentation
   (0) No brown spots
   (1) Uneven/some distinct brown spots

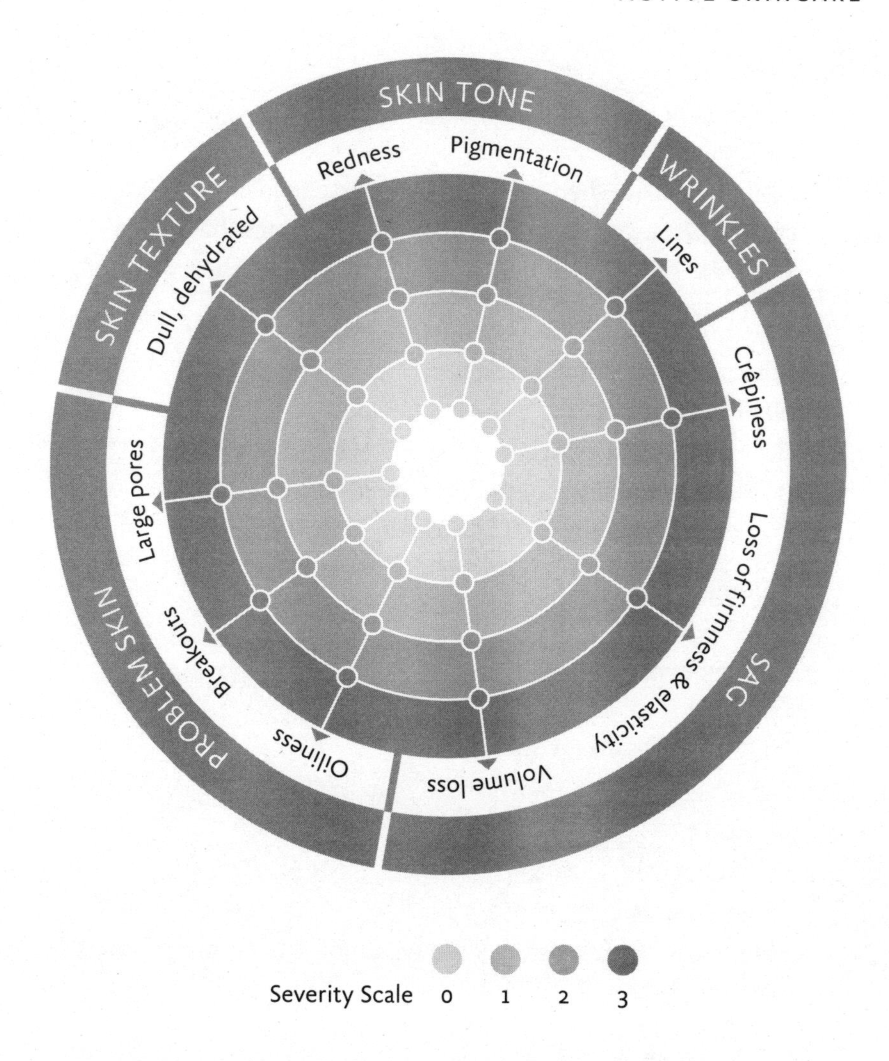

(2) Some patches, but they go away after the summer
(3) Brown patches that are always there

4. Lines
   (0) Line free!
   (1) Fine lines running horizontally across your forehead/ vertically between your eyebrows/crow's feet
   (2) Deeper wrinkles
   (3) I see wrinkles even when I am not moving my face

5. Crêpiness
   (0) None/plump hydrated skin
   (1) Fine lines under my eyes
   (2) Crows' feet when I'm not smiling/extended crows' feet
   (3) Not just eyes: 'accordion lines' (vertical lines that appear to the side of your mouth when you smile), 'barcode lines' (vertical lines that appear above your upper lip)

6. Loss of firmness and elasticity
   (0) Firm bouncy skin
   (1) Slower bounce back
   (2) Skin around my mouth is not as smooth
   (3) 'Droopy' downturned lips, 'down in the mouth'

7. Volume loss (no support, subcutis)
   (0) Lifted
   (1) Somewhat sagging
   (2) Saggy
   (3) Forming jowls on my jawline

8. Other issues: mark them on the same scale of 0 to 3.
   Oily skin
   Breakouts
   Large pores
   Milia (small bumps that look like whiteheads but don't go away)
   Dark circles
   Eye bags
   Upper eyelid drooping
   Barcode lines
   Thinning lips

Score Chart

DULL, DRY COMPLEXION		You should respond superbly to skincare, even just the basics. Start with the reset programme. You'll get quick wins by using acid exfoliants. Targeted ingredients: To hydrate: glycerin, squalene, urea. Plus anti-inflammatories: azelaic acid, zinc, niacinamide, feverfew, oats. Procedures to boost skincare: Medical facial, peels, mesotherapy, IPL (see Chapters 7 and 8)
REDNESS		Redness/flushing can be hugely improved with skincare. Start with the intervention programme. Targeted ingredients: Niacinamide, azelaic acid, salicylic acid for exfoliation. Procedures to boost skincare: Laser/IPL may be required for the final push (see Chapters 7 and 8).
PIGMENTATION		Wear sunscreen Start with the reset programme. Then pigmentation usually requires prescription skincare. Targeted ingredients: Vitamin C, niacinamide, kojic acid can help. Liquorice is a good ingredient if you have sensitive skin. Procedures to boost skincare: Laser/IPL may be required (see Optimize, Chapter 8).

WRINKLES		Start with the reset programme for mature skin. Include: antioxidants to boost defence: resveratrol, alpha-lipoic acid, CoQ10. Procedures to boost skincare: Injectables may be needed to see a significant improvement (see Optimize, Chapter 8).
SAGGING		Start with the reset for mature skin. But skincare is really just preventative here. A plumping effect can mask a loss of volume to an extent, but not significantly. Procedures to boost skincare: Skin boosters, fillers, threads, EBDs (see Regenerate and optimize, Chapters 7 and 8).
OTHER ISSUES		Use the index at the end of the book to find where I have dealt with these issues individually.

How much does it bother me? (GET HONEST!) (1 = very little/not often 3 = maybe once a day 5 = a lot/ think about it several times a day)	
DULL, DEHYDRATED COMPLEXION	
REDNESS	
PIGMENTATION	
WRINKLES	
SAGGING	
OTHER ISSUES	

What is your current skincare routine?

Based on the advice in this chapter, fill in your current routine and assess possible changes you could make so that you get the most out of your time and money.

PRIORITIES	AM	PM
Cleanser		
2nd cleanse (if/when required)		
Face cloth/muslin (Y/N)		
Toner		
Exfoliant		
Treatment (acne, pigment)		
Eye cream		
Serum		
Retinoid		
Moisturizer		
Sunscreen		
Other		
The time it takes		

	HOW OFTEN?
Masks	
Prescription products	
Facials	
Other cosmetic procedures	

CHAPTER ROUND-UP

- Be prepared to spend: time and money.
- It's a marathon, not a sprint. Slowly, slowly.
- Give your skin a break from all the products you've been using. All my programmes start with stripping back.
- Get your BASICS right. That means sunscreen every day, a gentle cleanser plus the 3 A's: vitamin A, acid exfoliant, ascorbic acid antioxidant.
- Remember, successful skincare should ALWAYS improve skin function as well as cosmetic appearance. That's what gives long-term results.

Chapter Five

Your consultation: a guide to aesthetics

If Chapter 2 was *'do or don't'*, here I will lay out *'do what, when'*. From now onwards in the book, we are moving along the PAP to where the clinic treatments start. You don't have to make a decision about whether these are right for you, right now. I want to give you all the information you need to make your own - informed - decision, whether you end up having one treatment, 10 or none.

In Chapter 2, I challenged you to look at your mindset, to ask yourself why you were reading this book and what kind of commitment you wanted to make to this positive ageing journey. For some of you, the answers may have come easily, but more likely, some soul-searching will have gone on.

Perhaps you've gone from, 'Why care? As a feminist, my worth is so much more than how I look,' to admitting that you have started to take a back seat at work and are confused as to why your self-confidence has started to dip. This is very common, and something, both as a doctor and as a client, that I have had to contend with too.

It is why, when I first meet with clients, we spend a large part of the initial consultation discussing wants, needs, expectations and fears. My approach is always to understand the person and their motivation before even talking about appearances and the result of any treatments. Treatments are about the surface, so they cannot change the mind.

Most people book in for a consultation in the clinic after years of thinking about it. A lot have seen the results of friends who've been, but haven't spoken about it to anyone. Some people look in the mirror one day and make a snap decision to come. Some know exactly what they want (or think they do), some don't, and others have been to different clinics and are not sure about the results they've had. My job is to recognize what will work on your face and what is worth doing, and to tell you the results you can expect. I tend to be conservative in the way I treat: it's always possible to do more later on if needed.

To start with, I am going to walk you through your first consultation, exactly how I would in my clinic. It's where my clients begin to understand more about their skin, get an overview of the treatments on offer, and learn how to get the best from them.

This is not a shopping list, and it is not the in-depth look at treatments that's coming up later in the book; this is a simplified explanation of what happens in the PAP if you decide it's right for you to go beyond skincare.

That said, if you want to jump in at the top of the PAP and start with treatments, it's completely up to you. And many people do. As a mother to three boys, I know that getting 8 hours of sleep every night has been an impossibility for a few years (maybe forever!), and I also know how hard it is to fit it all in: the gym, yoga, cooking, friends, sex, face massage! And then to also cut back on sugar and alcohol? I know from experience how much of a struggle this can be, so never feel guilty for your choices. All our lives are different and you deserve to feel happy in yourself, however you choose to do that.

However, as with most things in life, if your foundation is strong, you will reap better results. By which I mean that the treatments at the top of the PAP will have the most impact if your mindset is in a good place, your lifestyle is as healthy as you can feasibly make it and your skincare is tailored and effective. But remember, no one can do everything, and those who try often fail and give up! Pep talk over, let's get started . . .

Your assessment

Before you come into the clinic, you'll fill out a form about your mindset and your lifestyle, including further questions that delve into what you see when you look in the mirror, as well as the detailed skin analysis, below. This is a clinical tool that I review to give me a clear idea of the condition of your skin and how you feel about it, before I see you in person.

To do the analysis, you simply look in the mirror and grade your skin using the skinscore diagram below. You consider all its qualities, from texture and tone to volume, and grade each one from 0 (not a problem) to 3 (an issue you would like to address). Fill in your scores on the table below.

Even if you're not going into a clinic, this is useful. You can use it to measure how your skin responds to any skincare and lifestyle changes, as well as before and after treatments, if you choose to have them.

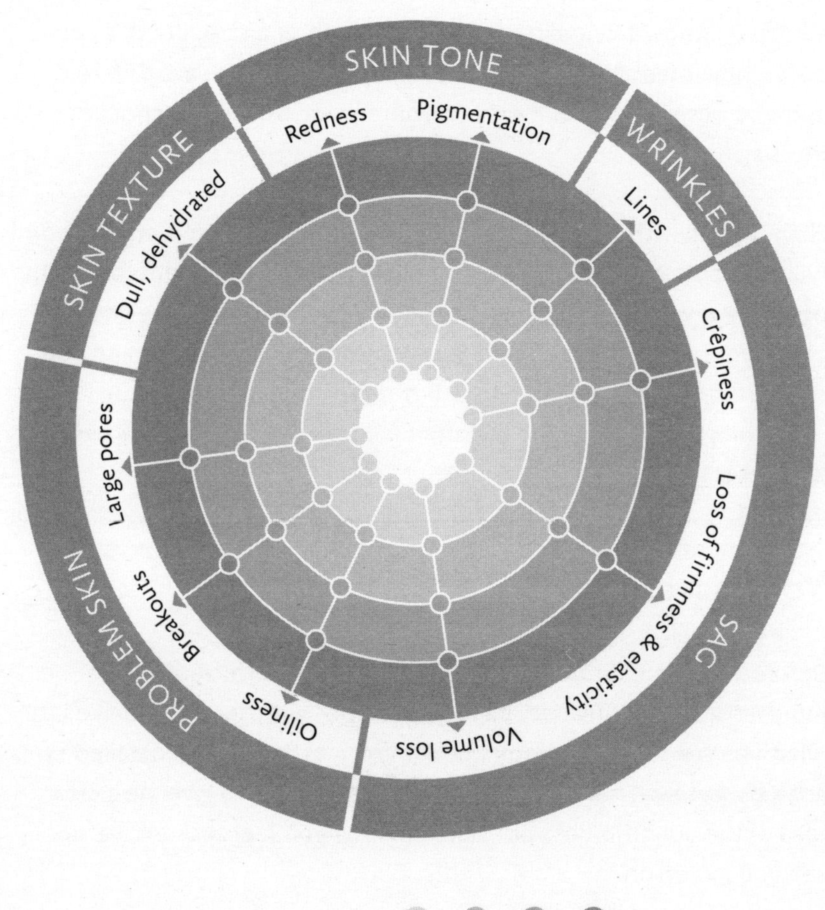

Severity Scale 0 1 2 3

	Score (0–3)	Concern? (0–3)
DULL, DEHYDRATED		
REDNESS		
PIGMENTATION		
WRINKLES		
CRÊPINESS		
LOSS OF FIRMNESS		
VOLUME LOSS		

	Score (0-3)	Concern? (0-3)
OILINESS		
BREAKOUTS		
LARGE PORES		
OTHER		

Static photos vs. the dynamic you - a doctor's perspective

Then, before meeting clients for the first time, I *always* take a good look at the series of photos taken at 'check-in', when you meet the front of house team. I study the proportions, angles and contours of the face. All of this, along with the diagram, helps inform me when drawing up an initial treatment plan in preparation for our first meeting.

However, when you walk in, and I shake your hand, and see your blink impression in that first split second, my priorities can shift. I might think to myself, nope, treating those deep forehead wrinkles is no longer going to have the greatest impact; she looks so much better smiling; let's volume replace and restore contours and proportions. How your face moves is absolutely key.

During that first meeting, we'll talk about your skin's whole history, including your current skin regimen as well as your past skin and aesthetic history (back to your teenage skin!), lifestyle factors, and your concerns and goals. Then I'll examine your skin manually and digitally. This might also include using software that zooms in to quantify issues such as pores or redness. Or it might be using probes that I put on to the skin to measure, for example, elasticity or sebum levels.

What you see vs. what I see

This is the most emotional part of the consultation. I ask people to really open up, to talk about their face and skin, what they put on the skin analysis but also how they feel. Is it easy to swing from liking your skin one day to hating it the next? Is there something that hasn't necessarily changed over time but the way you *see it* has?

It would be wrong to attempt to stay 100% objective, to stick to the assessment I made before I met you. I need to factor in your face in 360 degrees, while you are moving and talking and expressing. And, even more importantly, your perspective matters just as much as mine. How and what you feel about your appearance needs to be taken very seriously.

For example, if you tell me a particular feature is bothering you - under-eye circles, wrinkles, sagging, pigmentation - I will ask how often you think about it. If you're spending time every day applying layers of make-up to conceal it or try to compensate for it, perhaps it is time to treat it. That's the case even if I, as your doctor, don't see it as significant.

Conversely, if I were to focus solely on what the client sees and wants, to robotically treat that, it would also be a recipe for disaster. Because very often, clients will focus on a thing that has become an issue from years of analysing, possibly stemming from their teenage years. We all have our 'thing', it's completely normal, but it's my job to help you see past it.

How can you find out if what other people see is what you see? A straight-talking but good friend can be a great sounding-board. And looking at photographs of yourself works much better than looking in the mirror when trying to get an honest view. Although everybody sighs when they first see their clinic photo, when I sit with a client and talk through it, it does seem to encourage objectivity. Also, I often ask clients to show me pictures in which they like the way they look. This helps me to think about the features they are happy with and therefore what we should aim to enhance when we think about treatments.

Best bang for buck: your annual skin plan

OK, I know I have just bombarded you with information and it's only the first consultation! We are going to return later in the chapter to the specific treatments you may want to consider, but first I'll explain why you should aim to have an annual treatment plan, and what to consider in order to build one.

First, you need to know why it's a good idea. An annual plan is how you'll get the most value out of your time and money budget. Worked out between client and practitioner, it sets your expectations and avoids you either spending or doing more than you'd like, the slippery slope that so many people tell me they are nervous about. It gives any treatment the time it needs for the results to show, rather than you booking in for another one too soon.

Also, a plan means you'll never have to be tempted by any new 'miracle' product or treatment you hear about. As new ones come out, I monitor them, and I introduce them to the clinic when I'm convinced there is a place for them. There is no point in rushing into anything, just because it is new or getting press.

A year is a good period of time, as it allows you to focus on the skin issue or issues that are coming up for you. This is the absolute opposite of dabbling or chopping and changing, which your skin dislikes. Planning a year will give your skin time to heal and function at its best - this slow and steady approach, without doubt, gives the best results.

Now you have some decisions to make.

How much time can you spare?

Honestly, how much time are you prepared and able to spend on your regime, morning and night? How many appointments a year do you want in clinic? Some of my clients are super-keen to do as much as possible with skincare at home. Others much prefer regular visits to the clinic. At home, the basics will take you from 60 seconds to a maximum of 10 minutes, twice a day. Most clients have a monthly clinic appointment planned into their year, but some have more, and some have less. Be honest, how much time have you got?

How much downtime can you have?

As I said in the last chapter, introducing more active skincare ingredients, the ones that really work, such as chemical exfoliators and vitamin A, can unsettle your skin for a few weeks, make it drier, or you may have some breakouts or mild flushing. The same is true for some regenerative and optimization treatments; as we go through them in the following chapters, I'll describe any after-effects and how much downtime you may have. No downtime means you can go straight back to work or play, with nobody noticing a thing. Downtime can mean 30 minutes' flushing that can easily be covered with make-up, and the small bumps from injections that usually settle in 20 minutes to 1 week of swelling, redness and scabs. Or it can mean a few weeks when your skin is dry and irritated, as you adjust to a new, potent skincare programme. I'll tell you what you can expect as I describe each treatment.

Are you in a hurry?

For clients who want dramatic results sooner, I do sometimes agree to fast tracking. For some, that might be a 12-week clinical prescription skincare system such as Obagi Nu-Derm (see page 151), which works to treat mature skin as well as pigmentation. Be aware that with this kind of intense programme you are likely to experience significant dryness, flaking and irritation in the first few weeks. For others, I will go straight to the top of the pyramid to optimization treatments, such as BTX or fillers. But I want to say again, it is the slowly, slowly maintenance programme - of lifestyle change plus skincare plus the maintenance facials you're about to hear about in Chapter 6 - that will ultimately give you the stand-out results that will keep you looking naturally healthy and glowing through the years.

What's your budget?

How much are you really able to spend a month? You'll typically need to spend more in your 50s and beyond than you did in your 30s. Of course, there is huge flexibility here and I always ask how much clients are currently spending on their regime before discussing options.

Most clients come into clinic wanting a quick fix - the 'wow' effect - which may indeed *initially* seem like the best bang for buck. But, as I've already described, these don't necessarily have the longest-lasting effects. The aim is to spend wisely.

I always encourage people to consider treatments in the order of the PAP because the better your skin quality from lifestyle and skincare, the less you'll need of the more invasive, expensive treatments, and the longer the results last too. Out of all the other lifestyle changes I suggested in Chapter 3, two are no-brainers before you start spending serious money on treatments. The first is, do not smoke. Your skin hates it. You won't get the results you want from treatments, and the results you do see won't last. The second is, don't sunbathe, and always wear sunscreen, even in winter. This is especially true if you are treating pigmentation but it's true for all of the 5 signs of ageing.

When it comes to the cost of skincare, these are very rough estimates for someone who doesn't have a specific skin condition. You could buy the 5 basics of skincare from around £600 a year. That's from less expensive brands, for example The Ordinary or La Roche Posay, whose products vary from less than £10 to around £40. I'd advise spending a little more on your vitamin A (see page 128 for details). I know this amount may already sound a lot, but think about what you already spend. A recent survey showed that the average spend in the UK on skincare alone is £500 to £1,000 a year. Some of my clients have confessed to spending upwards of £3,000 a year, but it isn't necessary to fork out that much; you can buy good-quality products for less.

Below are the building blocks of what you can include in your annual plan, alongside your lifestyle medicine and skincare routine, of course. I'll go into what each treatment involves, including the exact price, time taken and downtime, in Chapters 6, 7 and 8.

As the prices of the treatments vary hugely, as does how often you'll need them, it's hard to assess what you might spend before you know the details. But to give you a ballpark figure, this is what people spend in the clinic.

- In your 30s, you might spend £1,800 per year. This would cover a combination of skincare, 3 maintenance facials, and 2 sessions of BTX.
- In your 40s, you might spend £4,000 a year. This is for skincare, 6 facials, 2 regenerative treatments, BTX and fillers.
- In your 50s and beyond, your spend might go as high as £6,000 a year. This would include the same as in your 40s but adding extra filler and regenerative treatments.

Where should you start?

This is the approach to building your programme that is most effective, following the order of the PAP:

Level 1: Maintenance: in-clinic facials including some non-invasive add-ons for radiance and skin health

There are usually 3 steps: cleanse, exfoliate, and treat/boost with active ingredients. That might sound similar to a high-street or cosmetic facial you'd have in a salon or at a spa, but maintenance facials are a significant step up from these in terms of their effect on skin. They involve not only strong active ingredients, but also a technological add-on, using tiny needles or a handpiece that infuses those ingredients in deeper, and also LED (see page 191). The idea is to boost skin's hydration, circulation and/or repair mechanisms.

Often in the clinic, we will combine a maintenance facial with a regeneration treatment, which I cover next. The purpose of these maintenance level treatments is to boost the impact of the ingredients you're using at home with your skincare. Then at home, your skincare should sustain the results of your facials.

Cost: From £95, depending on treatment.

How often? Most usually, from 3 to 12+ times a year, or when needed.

Level 2: Regeneration: Treatments that improve the tightness, plumpness and quality of the skin

This next level includes all treatments that trigger new collagen and elastin in your skin. These kinds of treatment are perfect for when a skin reset is needed, such as improving loss of elasticity or sagging. The principle of these treatments is to trigger a 'healing' response in your skin. This may sound strange, but the way to do this is via controlled damage, which prompts skin to heal itself. The fibroblasts wake up and start pumping out collagen, and the area is flooded with all the ingredients we need to make new skin. The damage can be done with little needles, such as medical microneedling or derma-rolling, or with 'skin boosters', which involves tiny, shallow injections of skin-boosting ingredients (such as hyaluronic acid) all over the face. Or with heat, using the energy produced by radio-frequency, ultrasound and laser treatments to trigger the healing response.

Cost: From £200 to £3,000, depending on the treatment. Details in Chapter 7.

How often? Most usually, a course of 3 to 6 treatments, once a year.

Level 3: Optimization: Treatments that change the contours and proportions of the face as well as resurfacing treatments that erase excessive pigment (red or brown) and smooth out skin texture and/or wrinkling

These are the cherry on top of the pyramid, the ones that can make an instant, visible change to your face. It might be BTX to soften wrinkles (see page 219). Or facial fillers used to address loss of structural support and facial volume (see page 222). This category also includes thread lifts, which is where suture threads are inserted to subtly tighten and lift parts of the face (see page 243). And it includes some lasers, used to treat deeper pigmentation (see page 242), as well as redness and wrinkles. I always suggest subtle tweaks, and a step-by-step programme rather than dramatic overhauls.

Cost: Varies hugely, but from £170.

How often? Varies hugely, depending on treatment. BTX, for example, is often every 4 to 6 months, but it can be longer. See Chapter 8 for specific treatments.

What does an annual plan look like?

These are as individual as the people who walk through the clinic doors. Now that you know all the factors to consider, you can start to decide what yours will look like, according to your skin, your budget and your time. Some people are more prone to redness in winter, some want their pigmentation treated after the summer months, so think about everything, from when you plan to go on holiday and how busy work will be, to when you have big expenses going out throughout the next year.

The lightest programme will be for someone who looks after their skin with skincare only. The next level might be skincare plus coming into the clinic every 2 months for a maintenance facial. And then some people have this, plus BTX twice a year. There is no right or wrong plan, so find the perfect one for you.

What treatments are right for you?

Now we come to thinking about your plan. As I said, there's usually a difference between what you see and what I see and how I would treat it . . . These are some of the most common issues I am presented with and how I'd approach them, ideally after both your skincare regime and maintenance facials are under way.

You see: Tired, sad, cross - 'I don't look how I feel'
What I see: We spend so much time examining our own faces and noticing things that might not stand out to other people. That is not to say you are wrong, but it's not the whole story.

There are objective metrics of beauty out there, dating back as far as Leonardo da Vinci, and they are a good starting point for me. But really, I want to make you look more like you, but a you that looks relaxed, and that makes you feel good. My aesthetic judgement centres on the overall, instant impression a face makes - the blink impression - because people see an awful lot without even focusing on a face.

There are plenty of techniques that can simply and oh-so-subtly tweak that impression. Smart BTX, for example, placed in tiny amounts at the tail of the eyebrow or around your jawline, can lift a tired or sad look but leave no tell-tale signs of treatment.

You see: Lines and wrinkles - 'This line reminds me of my mother'
What I see: Bah! Wrinkles do not have the impact you think they do. Far more important is uneven skin tone (brown and red) and volume loss (a 'flattening' in your mid-face that often starts in your late 30s). But, if a client is fixated, or sometimes if the lines are too distracting, it can be a place to treat, using fillers and/or BTX. For example, deep frown lines can make you look cross, or nose-to-mouth lines (nasolabial folds) can accentuate very early changes to the jowl area.

You see: Texture - dull, dry, rough, or crêpey
What I see: Poor light reflection. As described in Chapter 1, this is not only pretty much a universal problem post-35 but it's a quick win. Exfoliation is the answer. Chemical exfoliation is my preference over abrasive scrubs or brushes. That means a chemical acid leave-on exfoliator lotion toner as part of your skincare routine and a stronger peel added on to your maintenance facial. Well-exfoliated skin does not only look fresher, it will feel smoother, plumper, stronger. And all your products will penetrate so much better and more evenly. Win-win!

There's more detail on which exfoliators to choose in Chapter 4 and on which facials will help too in Chapter 6.

You see: Tone - brown spots and/or redness
What I see: Skin that needs protecting from the sun. As you already know, pigmentation or brown spots is your skin doing its job to protect you. When it perceives a threat, such as UV rays, it produces melanin - the pigment that gives you a tan. This is designed to act as a filter - protecting collagen and DNA that lies deeper - but unfortunately, the cells that produce melanin can become ultra-sensitive, with a very low threshold.

Around 80% of my clients are using a concealer to cover up all sorts of pigmentation and redness when they first come to see me, but gradually they stop over the course of their programme. That's what I love about aesthetic treatments, they give you the freedom of not wearing make-up. Unfortunately, eliminating pigmentation may not be possible and it's not quick. But there are some excellent skincare and programmes available (see page 151), and also increasingly sophisticated laser treatments that are more powerful, and need less downtime (see page 240). As for redness, one of our most popular treatments is a 5-minute laser that zaps red vessels around the nose and can last 6 to 12 months (see page 242).

You see: Sagging - from 'not as plump or firm' to 'slack skin or jowls'
What I see: Loss of firmness means a loss of elasticity (dermis), facial support (bone) and volume (fat), which then leads to sagging. Fillers have a bad reputation, but it absolutely is possible to reinvigorate a face without completely changing it.

When someone has had good work done, you cannot put your finger on what has changed. The goal is not to give someone cheeks they have never had, or to distort their natural face shape - don't start me on lips! - but to compensate for lost volume. To restore proportions, change light reflection - just like make-up can.

You see: 'My skin and face look OK - but I want to look my best at 40, 50 . . . 70'
What I see: Lots of great possibilities. Refreshingly, the most common request from clients is, how do I best take care of my skin and face from here? The starting point is always to talk you through the PAP and work out an annual treatment plan.

Now you've got some idea of the treatments you might be interested in having, you can start deciding on the building blocks of your PAP. Chapters 6, 7 and 8 will help you really work out what combination of things is going to work best in your annual plan.

CANCER

I'm seeing more and more women present to the clinic having been diagnosed with cancer. They tell me that there is so much conflicting advice out there and they are often being met with incredulity should they dare consider cosmetic intervention at a time when surely appearance *shouldn't* matter. But it *does*. There are safe products and treatments that do make a difference. It's time to spread the word - watch this space.

CHAPTER ROUND-UP

- Consider everything from skin texture and feel to volume, and grade it.
- What is your 'blink impression'?
- What you consider to be issues may not be. Because what you see in the mirror may not be what other people see.
- Start to think about whether you want to explore any treatments and what that might look like for you - I will explain them in more detail in the following chapters.
- Be real with yourself on what you can commit to financially and time-wise.
- Consider all treatment levels (Active Skincare, Maintenance Facials, Regenerative and Optimizing treatments) and start building an annual plan.
- No stress! Choose a routine and plan that you will enjoy!

Chapter Six

Maintenance facials

Welcome to the maintenance level of the PAP. This is the level if you want to achieve a bit more than skincare can do, but you're not up for cosmetic treatments. As you'll see, it's all about facials - but not as you know them. These facials are medical grade, customized to your skin, performed at an aesthetics clinic, using active skincare and with the help of customized machines or devices.

Beauty or high-street facials might do a great job to pamper and hydrate, but they have no real impact on skin biology or function; therefore, no profound effects, and you will enjoy a 5-day skin boost at best.

Medical facials address (and aim to correct) structural and functional changes of your skin as well as its appearance. They work at a cellular level, to slow down the processes of ageing, boost repair and regeneration. This shows as a lasting glow.

While the price of medical facials might feel like a serious investment to begin with, the benefits are huge and far outweigh the temporary boost you might experience with even regular high-street treatments.

The downside of medical facials is that there's no point in having one treatment. You can have a 'walk-in' appointment. But if you have chronic skin conditions or more advanced issues to address, it's better both to prep for at least 4 weeks, sometimes 12 weeks with skincare, and to have your facials as a planned part of your annual programme.

WHO IS IT FOR: If you want stand-out skin, medical facials are essential from the age of 35+ for improving texture (dry, dull skin), sensitivity and problem skin (oiliness, spots and pores).

They're good if you're looking to kick-start a skin renewal programme; to address skin changes seasonally or after life events - post baby, periods of stress, for example. And they're suitable for those with chronic skin conditions, where high-street facials can often exacerbate the issue.

They also give a kick-start boost if you usually have BTX and/or fillers but it's begun to feel as if they're no longer having much of an effect. They help reduce a mismatch between a smooth(er) forehead and possibly crêpey skin around the mouth. They're also a great way to make other results last longer. As a result, you won't be in such a rush to get back into the clinic when lines start reappearing if you have a background of clear, glowing skin.

Remember, though, if you decide to invest in a course of these facials, you can't expose your face to the sun. Medical facials stimulate the skin and so raise the risk of pigmentation, if you are prone to it. Unless you are wearing a daily sunscreen, they're pretty much a waste of time and money.

TIME: Express facials can be performed in 20 to 30 minutes, but the full version can last 45 to 60 minutes. As you'll see, they're often combined with the regenerative treatments described in Chapter 7 (mostly for convenience, as part of an annual plan). And many of my clients will

schedule them for immediately before their injectable appointments, detailed in Chapter 8, to save having two visits to the clinic.
DISCOMFORT: None. They might not feel pampering but they are pretty satisfying.
DOWNTIME: None. In fact the opposite: you will walk out with a glow.
RESULTS: After one treatment most people will enjoy a glow and clarity that lasts 10 days. After 3, you will be hooked, with results lasting a month or more.

As part of an annual plan, you'll usually have a maintenance facial every 4 to 12 weeks. The best time to have them is every skin cycle, i.e. 4 to 6 weeks. Everyone's skin cycle is different, but you will know when you need to have another session as you will most likely start using more make-up, either because you want more glow or you feel you need to conceal.

Alternatively, you can sign up for an intensive course to kick-start a treatment plan or to prepare for a big event. Intensive courses usually mean 3 or 4 facials every 10 to 14 days, ideally after having prepped with products for 4 weeks.

PRICE: What can you afford? As a guide, from your late 20s, you might have 3 to 6 facials a year (costing from £65 per facial). In your 40s, you'll have ideally 9 to 12 a year (from £65 to £165 per facial). If you start adding in regenerative treatments in the next chapter, prices can go up to £200. For some, monthly facials work best.

What does a facial involve?

Even when you've had a few treatments, it's important to have your skin assessed each time you come into the clinic. As clients come in regularly for facials, it's a good time to do this, and to tweak any homecare regime.

Facials follow three steps: cleanse, exfoliate and treat. If you're used to beauty facials, the 'treat' part will typically involve 'massage and moisturize', where the therapist will layer various serums, creams, masks and then perform lots of massage. The treat section, here, is more functional but also more effective.

1. Cleanse

We begin with advanced vacuum-assisted lymphatic drainage to help with the elimination of toxins that can accumulate in the skin. Then you should expect a very deep cleanse. In some medical facials, this stage is microdermabrasion, using tiny granules to take off the outer layer of dead skin cells. As with the physical scrubs we discussed in Chapter 4, this is too abrasive for most people's facial skin, especially if you suffer from redness or rosacea. I prefer hydradermabrasion, which uses water and a special vacuum tip to gently blast dirt, debris, make-up and pollution.

It doesn't matter how stellar your homecare regime is, you will be shocked when you see what has built up on your skin surface each time you have a medical facial (we usually collect it to show you!). Pollution, make-up, the accumulation of natural waste products from your own metabolism, are all removed. The resulting cleansed skin will allow your home skincare products to work better, as they won't have to work so hard to penetrate all those dead cells. Ultimately, this means you'll need less make-up.

2. Exfoliate

You can also expect a stronger exfoliation than your skincare will achieve. This has all the benefits of your regular acid exfoliant – both improving glow and, over time, the skin's function, but also prepares the skin for maximum benefits from the third 'treat' stage.

The exfoliation might be a peel or dermaplaning. A peel sounds harsher than it is, especially if you remember Samantha from *Sex and the City*'s terrible experience of redness and flakiness. It's just the name for chemical exfoliators, the same as the acids in skincare, except at a higher concentration. Different concentrations and acidities will be used depending on your skin and what you've been using at home.

Dermaplaning is using a blade to gently remove a build-up of dead skin cells at the skin surface. It gives a physical exfoliation with much less risk of damage than microdermabrasion. We may use dermaplaning before a peel, as it instantly allows the products that follow to be more effective as well as improving barrier structure and function.

3. Treat

This step involves active ingredients at higher concentrations than in skincare to actually treat a broader range of concerns. They might be vitamins, antioxidants, hyaluronic acid and skin-lightening ingredients for pigmentation, as mentioned in Chapter 4.

The therapist will use a medical device to get the ingredients into the skin for a better, longer-lasting result. That might be dermal infusion, using a handheld wand. Or to deliver the ingredients to just below the skin's surface, it might be superficial medical needling with tiny needles, or the mesogun, a handheld automated needling device. There's more explanation on how these work in Chapter 7 (see page 205). No anaesthetic is required for either, as they aren't painful, and the occasional red pinprick marks that are sometimes visible afterwards will settle within 24 hours.

The facial will be customized to what your skin needs. A common 'add-on' is LED (Light Emitting Diode) light therapy, using, most often, red or infrared light This stimulates the skin, supporting repair and regeneration.

Another add-on is cryostimulation. This involves having liquid nitrogen (aka dry ice) pumped all over your face for 2 to 3 minutes, which increases blood flow and makes the skin look instantly healthy and plump.

At this point in the facial, if you have milia, blood spots or skin tags, we can use a radio-frequency needle which uses heat to remove them. If you need extractions, we can use salicylic acid infusion to soften the dead material inside the pore, then a tiny vacuum to pull it out. This avoids the trauma that can come from manual extractions.

The facial will finish with sunscreen and, if necessary, a touch of make-up, a medical brand that allows your skin to breathe, such as Oxygenetix.

CASE STUDY

Treating pigmentation with skincare and facials

Sarah, 34, came to see me in the run-up to her wedding. She wanted a more even skin tone. She felt as if she had to wear make-up to cover up the pigmentation marks on her skin. This kind of dark spot issue is common in darker skin tones. It's called post-inflammatory hyperpigmentation (PIH), and it happens when breakouts cause a surge in melanin production as part of the skin's response to inflammation.

Sarah had pretty much given up treating her spots, as they'd been a problem for her for so long. This is why she didn't list this as her top concern. But without treating the underlying issue, there wasn't much point in treating the pigmentation. I noticed a higher number of dark spots around Sarah's chin area too. It turned out they were associated with plucking hairs, more inflammation that her skin was responding to by producing more melanin. I booked her in for a course of laser hair removal.

I upgraded Sarah's skincare to include prescription vitamin A and leave-on acid exfoliants (a combo of alpha and beta hydroxy acids). (For a similar skin treatment programme for adult acne, see page 154). These were both very well tolerated. She did report very mild sensitivity in the first 10 days, but it quickly settled completely. I also encouraged her to start using sunscreen daily. Black skin has a natural SPF of 13, so pigmentation is still triggered by UV.

Now that her skin had been tested by using these products at home, I had an understanding of how it would react to various ingredients at low concentrations. So she was ready for the higher concentrations used during medical facials in the clinic.

After 6 weeks of home skincare, I started Sarah on a course of medical facials and peels, to address her congestion and to brighten her skin. In the 4 months running up to her wedding, she went up a level, to 6 treatments in 4 months. By the time the wedding day came, Sarah was so pleased with the look of her skin: the pigmentation was hugely reduced, and her skin looked bright and pretty. Now, post-wedding, Sarah is having facials every 6 weeks, with home skincare tweaks for maintenance.

A step-by-step facial

This describes a typical medical facial for someone who has dry and dehydrated skin, using the brand I use, Hydrafacial. Other brands will be slightly different. It provides an intense hydration hit and light skin resurfacing, ideal for dry, dull, city-worn complexions, breakouts, acne, large pores or surface pigmentation. You'll leave the clinic with radiant, glowing skin and a clear complexion that is often immediate, peaking at

1 to 5 days and lasting at least a further 10 days. If you prep your skin prior to treatment with a complementary at-home skincare routine, or if you opt for regular treatment, results will certainly last longer - 4 to 6 weeks. This facial suits all skin types, including sensitive skins.

1. Assessment
2. Prep and cleanse
    - Advanced vacuum-assisted lymphatic drainage technique.
    - Double cleanse. The first is manual, with a short massage. The second is mechanical by hydradermabrasion, a nozzle that blasts water to gently lift dead skin cells.
3. Exfoliation
    - Exfoliation by hydradermabrasion. Using a specialized vortex tip which infuses skin with a tailored combination of alpha hydroxy acids (glycolic and salicylic acids). The exfoliation used can range from mild exfoliation for sensitive skins to a 'mini peel' for those with pigmentation/texture concerns.
4. Treatment
    - Extraction by hydradermabrasion. The water-jet's vacuum suction is a pain-free, hygienic way to dislodge dirt and clean out pores.
    - Antioxidant rejuvenation. Application of a personalized blend of skin-restoring antioxidants such as vitamins A and E, green tea and hyaluronic acid.
5. Soothe and hydrate
    - LED light therapy. A 20-minute session of non-invasive, tailored LED therapy that stimulates the skin's natural repair processes to boost overall health, plus reduce signs of ageing and sun damage.
    - Finish with an application of hydrating, protective moisturizer and breathable make-up if required - I use the Oxygenetix brand.

6. Skincare plan and next steps
   - If you don't already have skincare, you can receive your 12-week skincare plan to maximize your results at home.
   - Time commitment: 25 to 60 minutes (90 minutes to allow for skin consultation and imaging). For healthy skin maintenance, book in every 4 to 6 weeks. Cost: £165 (£95 for express).

ENERGY-BASED DEVICES (EBDs)

You often hear the word laser to describe all kinds of technologies: lasers but also light, LED and other machines. It's pretty confusing, as there are so many of these EBDs now on the market. The principle of all these technologies is that they push some kind of energy - light, radio-frequency, ultrasound - into the skin. This then triggers a 'wound-healing' response via controlled thermal (heat) injury. In the case of LED, it's a less extreme stimulatory process called photobiomodulation - which is why LED can be used by anyone, and you'll often find it in beauty clinics. I'll go into detail about all the other EBDs I use in later chapters, but LED is a great addition to a maintenance facial.

LEDs OR LIGHT EMITTING DIODES

These are suitable for every skin, as they involve no pain, no downtime and no risk. They can address multiple signs of skin ageing, from dull, dry skin to redness to brown spots and fine lines. The only downside is time, as LED needs to be done regularly for effect.

As well as having LED during a medical facial, you can have a stand-alone course (twice per week for 4 weeks) to give an immediate improvement on your skin that will continue for 8 to 12 weeks after completing the course. We also use LED post-procedure (needling, peels, laser), as it accelerates the result and reduces downtime.

The different wavelengths and colours of LED produce different effects:

- Red light: Anti-inflammatory. Stimulates new collagen production. Triggers healing at a mitochondrial level. It's been used by surgeons post-operatively for decades.
- Near infrared light: Travels deeper, improves collagen, elastin and hyaluronic acid levels. Also has a whole body effect, lowering cortisol and boosting serotonin. It's also very relaxing, as it feels as if you're lying on the beach! We also combine red and infrared.
- Blue light treats acne. It activates natural chemicals that destroy the cell membrane of P. acnes bacteria. For hormonal acne, alongside skincare, people find it useful to have 2 to 3 visits in the week pre-period.
- Green light regulates melanin production, which is helpful in maintaining an even tone if you are prone to pigmentation.

The beauty of peels

The days of the aggressive 'one-off' total peel that left you with a scabbed face are, thankfully, over. In fact, I've put peels into the maintenance section, as that's by far the most usual way for me to use them, during medical facials as a boost for dry, lacklustre skin.

You'll have met the main ingredients for peels already, in the skincare chapter, as they're a stronger version or a more concentrated form of acid exfoliants (see page 131). During the facial, they're applied with a gauze or brush, left to work, then neutralized (some peels self-neutralize). These chemical exfoliators are the workhorse of aesthetic medicine because they cover all the levels of the pyramid: skincare, maintenance, rejuvenation and optimization, depending on the ingredient(s) and how they are used. And they are good value.

My motto for peeling is low and slow. My view is, maintenance peels should not require time out of your schedule - just a few days when your skin may be a little dry, dull and/or flaky. Contrary to what most people think, you don't actually need to see visible peeling to achieve a fantastic result. Exfoliation is gradual - the treatment allows the dead skin cells of the epidermis to come away much more readily as you wash your face over several days post treatment. Used this way, they are a gentle effective alternative to the resurfacing lasers you'll meet in the next chapter. There are also peels to treat acne congestion, and some that include vitamin A.

Below, they are organized in terms of strength of the main peel ingredients, gentlest first. I tend not to use the strongest one, phenol peels. Some of the brands do have less strong home versions of the peels below, but my descriptions are of the clinic versions. Your clinician/ doctor will advise you about the best acid and brand to suit your skin.

- **Mandelic acid.** A great peel to have in summer. That doesn't mean you can go in the sun afterwards, but because the particles are larger, penetration is slower, which means less irritation. Less sensitized skin has a lower risk of any pigmentation issues. Try: Enerpeel MA.
- **Lactic acid.** This is my absolute favourite ingredient. It naturally has a lower pH and therefore you only need lower concentrations to get the same results as a glycolic peel - but without the side-effects. Try: Skin Therapy Repairing Exfoliant by Julia T. Hunter MD.

- **Salicylic acid.** This is the gold standard peel for acne. Most peel ingredients are water soluble, but SA is fat soluble and so is better able to penetrate the pores and skin that's producing high levels of sebum. Try: Epionce Sal-E.
- **Glycolic acid.** We do still use glycolic but it is relatively harsh and penetrates quickly, so it can cause inflammation. But it's also hydrating. Try: Neostrata, which is our go-to brand.
- **Retinol peels.** Retinol peels go deeper than most and can continue to penetrate 48 hours post-application. My favourite version of this is from Skin Therapy by Julia T. Hunter. It's important to prepare for this one with specific skincare, as well as barrier-strengthening ingredients for 12 weeks. Try: Neostrata Prosystem Retinol Peel or Professional Strength Peels by Julia T. Hunter MD.
- **TCA (trichloroacetic acid) peels.** Used for medium to deep peeling, these peels resurface and stimulate fibroblast activity and repair in the dermis. Good for the treatment of acne scarring. Try: Skin Tech Easy TCA, 4 lower concentration peels you have once a week, rather than one more intense treatment.
- **Phenol peels.** These are the deepest peels. They can achieve transformational results but you need to be in the hands of a doctor who performs them regularly; there are very few in the UK. This one does have downtime: 2 weeks at least. Try: Skin Tech Easy Phen.

WHO IS IT FOR: Age 25–70+. Peels are often used to treat dull skin as well as acne and congestion. In older skin, they'll treat pigmentation and wrinkles too. They're also good on the back and arms, for acne and 'chicken skin', aka keratosis pilaris. Peels aren't suitable if you like to tan your face, or you're about to go skiing or to the beach, however diligent you are with your sunscreen.
TIME: 15 to 30 minutes.

DISCOMFORT: During the application, 1 out of 3. It can range from a mild prickly feeling to the intense 20-second heat of salicylic acid.
DOWNTIME: Ranges from nothing up to a week (except for the phenol peel, see page 194) of redness and/or flakiness, depending on the ingredient(s) used.
RESULTS: Some acids give an instant glow, some take 10 days, some can take 4 weeks for maximal effect. The effects of deeper peels may even last a year. They're still included in some form in almost all my clients' treatment plans.
PRICE: From £65. Usually a course of 3 to 6 treatments, 2 to 4 weeks apart.

CASE STUDY

Dull, wrinkly skin after a baby

Jo, 38, came in asking for BTX to treat what she described as her 'crinkly' forehead. I didn't think this was the issue. Rather that her skin looked dull and ashy, which is often the case with darker skin. Jo told me she's of South Indian origin.

I asked about her skincare, and she told me she was using wipes to cleanse, and a whole range of expensive facial oils, serums and creams. I immediately banned wipes, and put her on an active skincare regime including the 5 basics you read about in Chapter 4. As she likes the ritual of massage, using a cleansing oil worked well for her. She followed this with the Julia T. Hunter MD skincare system, using Epionce barrier-supporting moisturizer as required, which was less as her skin condition improved. Over the next few weeks, I introduced a stronger acid exfoliant, then vitamin A.

Jo had her first medical facial a few days after her initial consultation, to kick-start her new regime and prepare her skin for her new products. Then she was on a programme of every

6 weeks. After a few months, she had a course of retinol peels too (see page 194). Jo's skin has completely lost its ashy tone, and it's plump and well hydrated. She looks really radiant. She is now in two minds whether even to have BTX at all.

The lowdown on beauty facials

Super facialists

In recent years a new breed of facialist has emerged, blurring the lines between high-street and clinical treatments. Practitioners such as Teresa Tarmey, Pamela Marshall, Joanne Evans and Dija Ayodele use the same principles and indeed the same ingredients and devices as clinics, but combine them with some old-school pampering in a luxurious setting.

These are excellent treatments. Always remember, the best results come if facials are part of a comprehensive aesthetic programme, so don't expect the same results from a one-off.

Microcurrents

Microcurrent machines are used in facials to 'work out' the muscles of the face and temporarily tighten and lift skin appearance. They've been around for decades and are now becoming more and more popular as home microcurrent devices - examples of brands you might have heard of are Nuface and Ziip. I am happy for my clients to enjoy the effects, but the lift in skin *appearance* is temporary, a fast-track, very intense massage. For longer-lasting results you need energy or heat to target the dermis, contract and remodel collagen and elastin fibres and stimulate new skin regeneration. You'll find more information on regenerative treatments that do this in the next chapter.

Massage facials

Lately a new type of beauty facial has appeared on the high street, driven by companies such as Face Gym, that combine massage and dermal infusions. These really stand out.

Massage relaxes muscles and improves blood circulation, and therefore oxygen and nutrient supply to the skin. When skin is well hydrated and nourished it will have better function, and look more plump and revitalized. Massage also boosts lymphatic drainage. Lymph is a fluid that flows in a system of vessels all over the body, separate from blood vessels. It carries waste, toxins and excess fluid away from our tissues, depuffing and reducing fluid retention. This is super important in rosacea.

However, for cumulative, functional (not just cosmetic) benefits, massage needs to be done regularly. And pulling and/or tugging your skin hard is not a good thing, long-term. You can give yourself the massage and lymph benefits at home, by following the instructions in the box, using your own skin cleanser, balm or oil.

This is where the mindfulness of me-time and the ritual of skincare can really benefit you too. If you like accessories, there are plenty to choose from: gua sha, jade roller, Sarah Chapman roller, ice rollers for puffiness, but you can also just use your fingers and oils - whatever works for you.

A QUICK FACIAL MASSAGE TECHNIQUE

After applying a cleansing balm or oil:

1. Wake up your lymph, your body's waste disposal system.
    - Using the pads of your fingertips, apply pressure behind your ears, slowly stroke downwards toward the collarbone. Repeat 3 times.

- Apply pressure just under your chin with both thumbs and stroke towards the ears, running just below the jawbone. Repeat 3 times.
- Be gentle around your eyes. Place your fingers (minus your little fingers) under your eyes, on the orbit bone, with index fingers at their outer edge and ring fingers closer to your nose. Apply pressure, hold for a count of 5, then release. Repeat 3 times. Very light, brisk tapping over the orbit bone, using index and middle fingers and moving from side to side, is also an option here.

2. Reduce muscle tension.
   - Frown muscles. Place your fingers between your eyebrows (vertically), press firmly, hold for a count of 5, then release. Move both hands in small steps out towards your temples, repeat. Working from the middle of the forehead out, finish at your temples. Repeat 3 times.
   - Jaw clenching. Apply deep circular pressure at the angle of the jaw (without pulling on the skin) for 10 seconds minimum, but if there is tension there, for as long as you've got!
   - Chin. Thumbs under your chin, use your pointing fingers alternately to rub downwards vigorously, for 10 seconds minimum.
   - Jawline. Put thumbs under your chin with fingers fanned out on top. Press, hold for a count of 5, then release. Move fingers up and out slightly and repeat. Continue working along the jawline and finish right under the ears. Repeat 3 times.
3. Stimulate blood flow. Using sweeping upward movements, follow the contour of your jawline and cheeks. Repeat 5 times - but longer if you have the time.

Introducing regenerative add-ons

Whereas steps 1 and 2 (cleanse and exfoliate) of a medical facial are essential maintenance at every age, the third step (treat) will vary. As you age and depending on your skin, the treat part of the facial is likely to contain one of the regenerative treatments that are explained in the next chapter.

CHAPTER ROUND-UP

- Not all facials are created equal. Medical facials are targeted and results-based.
- An investment in time, money and patience is required. For maximum benefit, medical facials need to be part of a programme.
- Detailed skin assessments will benefit your home skin regime.
- Regular medical facials mean you'll need less make-up - either to give a glow or to conceal blemishes.

Chapter Seven

Regenerative treatments

These treatments are all about improving skin from deep down rather than, forgive the pun, papering over the cracks. This is about taking skin to the next level: in quality but in terms of the PAP, too.

The principle of regenerative treatments is to damage skin in a controlled and almost invisible way, in order to trigger a repair cascade and stimulate skin's regenerative processes, especially new collagen production. The result is not only that the skin's function improves but you see visible improvements in texture, so the skin looks more radiant, smoother, firmer, more supple and dewy. These treatments can also improve skin clarity and tone, reducing redness and pigmentation, and increasing skin's elasticity and bounce, and density, for less pronounced wrinkles, crêpiness and sagging as well as plumper-looking skin.

While the procedures are not usually painful, they're not pampering either. The controlled damage is done with heat in the case of energy based devices (EBDs), for example radio-frequency, ultrasound and lasers. In the case of medical needling, it's done with needles. Then there are treatments such as mesotherapy that use needles but also introduce skincare ingredients, 'skin boosters' such as vitamin cocktails or hyaluronic acid (e.g. Profhilo) or PRP (the 'Vampire Facelift') that trigger a response too. PRP ingredients are extracted from your blood, rather than being synthetic (see page 206). There's a lot of crossover in the second two categories, needling and skin boosters, which will become clear when we go into the treatments in detail.

Are these treatments for you?

Who benefits most from these treatments? I almost never recommend most of them until the age of 35, some of them not until 40. In your 30s you are not likely to see huge impact from these treatments - or at least it will be so subtle that your friends are not likely to notice any change. That said, some of the treatments can be an investment at this age, as long as you get good advice, stimulating just enough to trigger a positive long-term response, but not too much inflammation. I've pointed out a rough age limit for each treatment. But, for all of these treatments, from your 40s onwards, you will most definitely notice the pay-off.

You'll need to book in for a course to see real results, then have regular booster treatments, so they are quite a commitment in terms of time and money. As always, good skincare and maintenance facials should come first. Sometimes, if you're on a lower budget, you might choose to have facials and aesthetic injections such as BTX (see Chapter 8) but leave out regenerative treatments. But if you have the option, regenerative treatments are good combined with injectables, as they will make, for example, BTX treatments look good for longer, or allow for lower doses to be used, or for your dose not to need to increase over time. Regenerative treatments can also take away some of the contrast between a smooth upper face and a less smooth lower face that you might get if you only have BTX.

Smokers don't see great results with regenerative treatments. And, as before, if you are going to expose your skin to the sun you need to be very careful with the timing of these treatments. As they stimulate skin, your threshold to UV damage will be lowered. Be especially careful not to book in before skiing and sailing, as these make high levels of UV exposure practically unavoidable. If you are actively going to tan your face, these treatments will at best be a waste of time and at worst accelerate signs of ageing, especially pigmentation.

But regenerative treatments are good if you want to go up to the next level in keeping your skin looking fresher and firmer. Also, for those whose regular injectables are not lasting as long as they used to or not giving the same desired 'wow' results; and if you have new concerns to address, for example crêpiness and/or sag.

Some of the machines needed for these treatments are extremely expensive, so that is why the treatments are too. But the cost will also depend on who is performing the treatment, for example whether it's a therapist, medical aesthetician, nurse or doctor, and whether you're going to a beauty salon or a clinic. The trend is to combine one or two of these treatments for best results, as well as, for example, BTX, and that will put up the cost significantly.

The downtime of each treatment will vary too. Some treatments have none – people have radio-frequency on the day of a big event for an instant lift and glow, for example – but with others there can be some redness on the day, and dry skin at day 4. At the very worst you might experience redness that looks like comedy sunburn for 48 hours and then some tightness or flaking at days 4–5.

All these treatments are designed for the face, neck and chest, and I've mentioned the other areas they treat too, when relevant. Where possible, I usually combine these treatments with the maintenance facials in Chapter 6. This is to save clients coming into the clinic twice, but also the facial will allow you to get the most out of each treatment. The timings and prices given are for the treatment alone, not including the cost of the medical facial.

Which regenerative treatment is right for you?

Medical needling: collagen induction therapy

In this treatment, also often called dermarolling, the practitioner uses tiny needles to create micro-injuries, which then induces a controlled wound-healing response in the dermis and the production of new collagen type 1. There are 7 types of collagen but type 1 makes up 80% of the dermis and is the one hit hard by UV rays. Needling also increases skin thickness and moisture levels.

Medical needling can be done with a roller or needling pen. I prefer to use a pen, specifically the SkinPen, though there are other brands such as DermaPen. The SkinPen is FDA approved (that is, the US regulatory authority). It has a needle pad at the tip of a handheld pen, holding 11 needles that oscillate 120 times per second. I find that, compared to a roller, there's less tug as you move the device across the skin. There is also more precision when adjusting the needle depth, important for the different thicknesses of skin as you go around the face.

WHO IS IT FOR: Age 35+. Dull, dry skin. Slightly deeper wrinkles. Sagging. Visible pores. Acne scarring (not for active acne). Stretch marks.
TIME: 30 to 60 minutes.
DISCOMFORT: 2 out of 3. It can be performed without anaesthetic on the hardy. Moderate stinging or burning depending on the depth and intensity. For acne scarring or going deeper, anaesthetic definitely required.
DOWNTIME: Depends on depth. 0 to 4 days of redness and flaking.
RESULTS: A fantastic treatment that wakes skin up, addressing all the signs of ageing. I have seen improvements even in the most damaged, acne-scarred skin, although for this effect you will need a deep treatment that involves more downtime. For best results, prep skin by using vitamin A for a minimum of 6 weeks before the treatment.

People like needling as it's natural - i.e. it doesn't involve anything being injected. That said, I do like to combine needling with solutions that take it a step further than just the mechanical boost to skin. I might add mesotherapy (see page 205) to introduce peptide and vitamin cocktails. Or PRP (platelet rich plasma - see page 206). Or brightening agents, such as kojic acid or tranexamic acid, to treat pigmentation. For more severe sun damage (for example on the décolletage) I combine needling with hyaluronic acid skin boosters such as Profhilo (see page 208), sometimes in the same session, sometimes in alternate sessions.
PRICE: You should definitely have a course, rather than a one-off. Have 3 to 6 treatments, 4 to 6 weeks apart. Then repeat every 1 to 2 years. From £200 for a single treatment.

A WORD ON NEEDLING AT HOME

I've seen a lot of clients who bought their own dermarollers to do this during lockdown, and swore by it. However, I advise extreme caution. I am not a fan. Needling at home may help your skincare penetrate better - but are they the right products? Are the products you've chosen designed to be more effective at a deeper level? Are you sure they're not causing inflammation?

I also worry about long-term damage - tearing and chronic inflammation - from regular use of the roller, and in particular from needles that are blunt rather than medical grade. And finally, no matter how hard you try, at home you will find it almost impossible to replicate the hygiene levels of a clinic. I do think this is a case where a professional knows best.

Mesotherapy

This is a combination of very light needling and the application of products via needles to get ingredients deeper than if they're applied topically. That can be a bespoke cocktail of vitamins, minerals, enzymes, antioxidants and amino acids, depending on your needs. The aim is to rejuvenate and tighten skin. The advantage over medical needling is that product is injected into the skin rather than being pushed in by the needling process - the delivery is neater and so involves less waste. It's also less painful and has close to no downtime, especially if performed with a 'mesogun' rather than manually.

The depth of injection can be varied: either very superficial at 1mm, or 2mm which is called nappage, or deeper at 4mm. We usually combine a first pass of deeper injections to deposit the ingredients, then a more superficial layer of injections to stimulate the skin mechanically.

The idea behind mesotherapy is that it instantly boosts circulation and hydration, as well as stimulating the skin's metabolism for a longer-term boost in collagen and elastin production. It's popular post-summer using a cocktail of vitamin C and moisturizing HA to rehydrate and repair skin. You can also use this technique to administer PRP (see page 206).

WHO IS IT FOR: Age 30+. You will get some tightening from the needling but not as much as with the SkinPen, so it's better for younger skins or for maintenance. Good for delaying wrinkles and sagging. Brilliant for giving glow back to dehydrated skin.
TIME: 30 to 45 minutes.
DISCOMFORT: 1 out of 3. People describe it as prickly, scratchy and tolerable. No anaesthetic required.
DOWNTIME: None, just a slight flush.
RESULTS: A glow at 48 hours after treatment. It's a great treatment in your 30s. But a little bit of an indulgence in your 40s unless you're

using it as a delivery method for more potent ingredients, for example PRP (see below).

PRICE: £200 per session. Have 2 treatments, 1 to 2 weeks apart, then a third treatment 4 weeks later. Then do it regularly as part of a programme, but it's safe to do every 4 to 6 weeks.

PRP – aka 'The Vampire Lift'

The principle of this treatment is to use growth-promoting elements of your own blood – growth factors – to stimulate the production of new, youthful skin. The treatment involves taking a small amount of blood from a vein in your arm. It's then spun in a centrifuge to separate out the part of the blood that's rich in platelets and so in growth factors.

The treatment is known as PRP, short for platelet-rich plasma. The machine we use creates PRGF, short for Plasma Rich Growth Factor, because some studies show that PRGF has a slightly higher concentration of growth factors. 10ml of blood will give you 2ml of clear platelet-rich solution. The PRGF is then injected back into your skin. This can be manually with a syringe, or using a mesogun. Or it can be 'needled in' with a SkinPen.

Once in the skin, the PRGF has been shown to improve wound-healing mechanisms by stimulating skin regeneration, including increased activity of fibroblasts, increased levels of pro-collagen type 1 plus other growth factors, and better resistance to damage after UV exposure.

It's not only all natural but it's a powerful way to harness your body's own healing capacities and it addresses all 5 signs of ageing – what's not to love? It's true that there is still not much high-quality research on results in the aesthetic space, but it's been used in sports medicines for injuries and in dentistry to support implants for a long time. I've seen good results on the chest and hands too, but it's best combined with other treatments, which can get expensive. For the chest, combine with skin boosters (see page 208). For the hands, combine with fillers (see page 222) and IPL (see page 242) for brown spots.

WHO IS IT FOR: Age 40+. Very good for dull/dehydrated skin. Also treats redness, pigmentation, wrinkles and sagging.
TIME: 45 to 60 minutes.
DISCOMFORT: 1 out of 3 using a mesogun, 2 using the SkinPen or syringe.
DOWNTIME: Slight flush only if using a mesogun. One day of redness if needling, also needle marks for up to 48 hours and possible bruising. I prefer the mesogun.
RESULTS: Gives a glow from 48 hours after treatment, with best results at 4 to 6 weeks.
PRICE: From £650 for a single treatment. Have 3 to 6 treatments, 4 to 6 weeks apart. Then repeat every 1 to 2 years.

Aquagold

Dubbed the gold microinfusion facial, Aquagold is a type of mesotherapy with plenty of celebrity endorsement in the US. The handheld device contains 20 tiny gold needles to stamp the skin and deliver a tailored serum deep into your skin, stimulating collagen production and improving skin texture.

It's the serum that is the most exciting part of Aquagold. It can be customized to include vitamins and hyaluronic acid as well as PRP (see page 206) and filler and BTX, depending on your skin concern. This is a fantastic treatment for those who like going make-up free. It improves dewiness, fine lines, pores. It also evens out skin tone, both redness from flushing and rosacea as well as pigmentation.

WHO IS IT FOR: Age 40+. Expensive but effective, this is the queen of needling treatments, giving skin an extra bright, plump and polished look.
TIME: 30 minutes for the actual treatment. One hour including blood draw and anaesthetic.

DISCOMFORT: 1 out of 3.
DOWNTIME: Slight flush on the day. We recommend that you don't use make-up until the following morning.
RESULTS: Seen within 4 to 7 days. It really does give a beautiful light touch to the skin. The full combination - PRP, BTX and filler - is often reserved for special occasions, as it's £1,000. But there is a less expensive filler and BTX combination that's very good for crêpey necks and wrinkly foreheads, especially when traditional use of BTX is no longer appropriate; there's more about this on page 222.
PRICE: £600 to £1,000 as a one-off treatment. Depending on the solution used, results will last 2 to 6 months.

Hyaluronic acid skin boosters

These are shallow injections of hyaluronic acid (HA) that act like an inner moisturizer. HA is a fantastic humectant, produced naturally in the skin, but levels deplete as we age. What can be confusing is that filler injections are made of HA too. But you can't change contours or fill lines with skin boosters; they're not thick enough. Rather, skin boosters spread under the skin, hydrating, giving back bounce and smoothing it out.

Skin boosters are not a new concept but they're a hot one - with lots of new entries to the market. While Restylane Vital was the earliest one (in 2005), Profhilo is a current favourite at my clinic. It takes only 10 injections to cover the whole face, and another 10 if you want to treat the neck too. You may well see benefits within just 1 week as the HA droplets draw moisture into the dermis. The product breaks down within a month, then the longer-lasting impact (biorevitalization) kicks in, stimulating new collagen and elastin production. A second treatment at 4 weeks is often required to ensure that this process really takes hold, which should then give you 6 months of benefits on the face, and at least 4 months on the neck. There is nothing better on the market at the moment for early crêpey changes on your neck, the ones you notice when you turn your head from side to side. Same goes for the accordion lines when you smile wide, or for early volume changes around the mouth and chin. I prefer to use products with less 'spreading power', such as 'RHA1' or viscoderm, for barcode lines - the vertical lines above the top lip.

WHO IS IT FOR: Age 40+. Excellent for dry and dehydrated skin. Does plump the skin, so lessens wrinkles and lifts sagging a little. Excellent for crêpey neck. Other places I use it are on loose belly skin, and knees and elbows, as well as face and neck.
TIME: 15 minutes.
DISCOMFORT: 2 to 3 out of 3, depending on the brand used. Profhilo is the most painful, taking 10 injections each for the face, neck and chest. Each injection feels like a bee-sting and smarts for around 15 seconds. You will walk out with visible bumps that are difficult to cover or disguise. These usually last just a few hours on the face, but can take up to 3 days to completely settle on the neck and décolletage. Bruising and puffiness are also possible but not common.
DOWNTIME: Bumps under the skin, for from 3 hours to 3 days.
RESULTS: Depending on product, from 4 to 10 months. Almost everyone from the early 40s onwards will benefit. It gives a fantastic boost to your skin, hydrating it as well as plumping it and improving elasticity. Basically a bang for buck issue - for some it will be more of an indulgence. Also a great option before you move on to fillers, or if you want just a bit of smoothing out rather than a change in face shape.
PRICE: From £390 per treatment. Profhilo may need to be repeated 1 month later, as we encourage a double treatment the first time. Then regular treatments every 4 to 6 months. Many of my clients have single treatments every 4 months along with their injectable fillers.

Laser

There are quite a few lasers on the market that are used for skin rejuvenation. I use Laser Genesis ('Gen-V'), a fractional non-ablative laser, an approach that allows the skin to heal quickly. Another brand with similar technology is called ClearLift. These lasers are designed for the treatment of mild wrinkles, fine lines, photo damage, uneven skin tone and mild skin laxity, as well as pore refinement. But beyond the almost immediate benefits, which are often similar to chemical peels, the goal is also to stimulate new collagen production, while remodelling and improving the structure and function of existing collagen. The advantage of these lasers over peels is that there's no downtime.

WHO IS IT FOR: Age 30+. As well as the face, good on the décolletage. This is a treatment I like to combine with peels and/or skin boosters, including PRP (see also above).
TIME: 30 minutes.
DISCOMFORT: 1 out of 3. It feels like mild heat.
DOWNTIME: None.
RESULTS: Results are instant, especially skin-brightening and reducing redness. After the age of 45, you may not see such an immediate 'wow' as you leave the clinic, and results on redness won't last as long as IPL, so it may not be the best value. But there is no downtime and it's a good stand-alone option if you have reservations about chemical peels.
PRICE: £200 per treatment.

Radio-frequency (RF)

During a treatment, a handheld gun pushes energy deep into the skin, heating it to between 38 and 40°C. This gently stimulates dermal activity and kick-starts the skin's production of new collagen. It's mainly used for tightening and lifting the contours of the face, but it also leaves skin glowing. The whole face can be treated in around 30 minutes, there is no downtime – which is why RF is popular before big events – and the results last between 4 and 6 weeks.

WHO IS IT FOR: Age 35+.
TIME: 30 to 45 minutes.

DISCOMFORT: Between 0 and 1 out of 3. Most people say it's relaxing, like a hot stone massage, although occasionally, in some spots, it can feel too hot.
DOWNTIME: None.
RESULTS: It gives an instant glow and a lift that stays for weeks, even with a single treatment. It's an amazing instant pick-me-up, with visible results comparable to a brilliant facial massage - but lasting for weeks rather than days. Because the heat stimulates collagen remodelling and activates fibroblast, there will be ongoing structural and functional improvements in your skin that last even longer.
PRICE: £240. For best results, have 3 to 6 treatments, 4 to 6 weeks apart. Then either have regular booster treatment or repeat the course every 1 to 2 years.

RF microneedling

This is a step up from the usual RF treatment, great for improving skin firmness by addressing skin laxity as well as changes in skin texture. The machine we use is called Morpheus 8, and it beams skin with RF energy delivered via coated needles. This takes the energy deep into the skin, leading to subdermal fat tissue remodelling as well as contraction of dermis and new collagen, elastin and blood vessel formation.

WHO IS IT FOR: Age 45+.
TIME: 45 minutes.
DISCOMFORT: 2 out of 3 - anaesthetic is required.
DOWNTIME: Minimal. You may bruise and will have redness and a small grid of black dots for 72 hours, depending on the strength of treatment and the area treated; the neck and décolletage may be more sensitive. If you want to go lighter, you'll need a longer course, of 2 to 3 treatments, 6 weeks apart.
RESULTS: An all-round skin tightener. This can be a great treatment for early sagging in the lower face, jowls and neck.
PRICE: From £800 per session. A course of 2-3 ideally, then wait a year before repeating.

CASE STUDY

Going make-up free

Karen, 47, has been coming into the clinic to see me 2 or 3 times a year for 12 years. She typically comes before the summer and Christmas holidays. In her working life she's a barrister, so she spends her days completely coiffed and made-up. She doesn't like wearing make-up during her downtime, so what she wants from treatment is for her skin to look clear and healthy so she can go bare-faced.

I'd describe Karen's complexion as classic peaches and cream, very delicate. Her skin still looks plump and it has a glow. She's religious about skincare and wearing sunscreen daily, which is why it's stayed that way. She's also pretty disciplined when it comes to lifestyle; her working life can be very stressful, so she knows she needs to keep on top of stress, eat well and make sure she goes to bed early enough.

A fortnight or so before each holiday, Karen will have a radio-frequency treatment to stimulate collagen production in her skin, to give her quick lift and glow. She might also have skin boosters, specifically Profhilo, to smooth her skin. Especially pre-sun and sea, this helps stop the skin looking dehydrated, as well as plumping. She only needs a tiny amount of BTX in the lines between her brows and around her eyes because her skin looks so fresh. Karen tells me that once she's had her lashes tinted at the beautician, she is ready for her holiday. She absolutely loves not feeling the need to put on any make-up until she goes back to work.

Microfocused ultrasound (MFU)

This is the most exciting technology for skin tightening. It's delivered to both skin and SMAS layers (the fibrous tissue that connects facial muscles to the dermis and is lifted and stitched in surgery), so it can both tighten and lift. The brands you might have heard of are: Ultherapy, Ultraformer or Ultracel.

The principle is similar to radio-frequency in that it induces heat to create controlled damage in the deep dermis and subcutis, while leaving the overlying skin untouched. It increases cellular turnover and triggers new collagen production, so plumping, tightening and smoothing out fine lines and wrinkles.

There are downsides. It is expensive because the machine is expensive to use. Results aren't as consistent or predictable as BTX and fillers. Discuss expectations with your practitioner, as the amazing before/after pics may not necessarily apply to you. For every brilliant result, there will be 10 clients who are not blown away, so client selection is key.

Results also likely depend on the skill of the practitioner. They need to constantly adjust the treatment while visualizing skin layers, as the depth to focus the ultrasound power varies from client to client and in different areas of the face.

Because of the high price tag, it's been wrongly sold as a one-off or optimization treatment. But I prefer to see this as a regeneration and investment treatment. It does need to be repeated regularly.

WHO IS IT FOR: Age 45+.
TIME: 60 minutes.
DISCOMFORT: 2 to 3 out of 3. It's been toned down since it was launched, as it was too painful for most at optimal strength.
DOWNTIME: Usually none. Occasional swelling.
RESULTS: Impressive - if you are a suitable candidate. Smoother, tighter skin from 12 weeks post-procedure.
PRICE: From £500 for small areas, for example brow lift. £2,000+ for face. It's recommended to have an annual treatment.

Tixel

I've put Tixel in the regenerative section, but it fits here and also in the next chapter, Optimizing. This is another treatment that induces damage in order to promote collagen. Each 'shot' of energy fired through the handpiece creates multiple micro-channels in your skin. This then stimulates a healing response from the surrounding healthy, untreated skin.

Tixel can be used at low energy with similar results to the ClearLift or Gen-V laser treatment mentioned above. But when used at higher strength, it actually resurfaces the skin as well as stimulating it. This is what I'd call an optimization treatment, as it's especially good at treating roughness and fine wrinkles, such as under the eye, extended crows' feet that go down the cheek, or the 'bar code' wrinkles that appear around the mouth.

WHO IS IT FOR: Age 40+.
TIME: 20 to 30 minutes.
DISCOMFORT: 1 to 2 out of 3. If you go high strength, you'll need an anaesthetic.
DOWNTIME: There is downtime if you go high strength: black dots and swelling for 3 to 4 days. If not, there is none.
RESULTS: 2 to 3 repeat sessions required every 6 to 8 weeks.
PRICE: From £400 (eyes only) to £1,000 (full face), for a stronger treatment.

A QUICK GUIDE TO FACIAL ADD-ONS

We often combine regenerative (and optimizing) treatments with maintenance facials – for best results but also convenience and bang for buck! This takes careful planning, though, and a thorough consultation beforehand.

DULL, DRYNESS	1. Exfoliate: peel/hydradermabrasion/ dermaplaning 2. Hydrate: medical facial/dermal infusion, superficial needling, mesotherapy 3. Soothe: LED
REDNESS	Gen-V laser, IPL,* LED
PIGMENTATION	IPL
WRINKLES	Microneedling, mesotherapy, Aquagold
SAG	Skinboosters, RF skin tightening
BLACKHEADS	Extraction by hydradermabrasion +/- manual
MILIA	RF needling
PORES	Extractions, needling, Aquagold, BTX*
	IPL and BTX are optimizing treatements, covered in the next chapter

CHAPTER ROUND-UP

- To make sure you're getting best value for money, only move on to regenerative treatments once you have committed to regular active skincare and maintenance facials.
- The principle of regenerative treatments is that they improve skin from deep down and so slow down the ageing process.
- Be wary of a quick fix! They don't exist.
- They are not necessary for the next step - optimization - but they will help you get the best results.

Chapter Eight

Optimizing treatments

People come to me expecting BTX to work like a pencil rubber, to erase the lines on their face. When I tell them that it only softens lines, that it takes time and a holistic approach of skincare and treatments to help skin heal fully, there's often a mixture of disappointment and relief.

I explain that you could erase all lines, if you used enough BTX and fillers early enough, but that's the opposite of what I do. Because it would also erase all your personality, would leave you looking like a waxwork. I do not believe in changing someone's face. I never want to get rid of a person's ability to express their feelings.

Great work should enhance a client's innate beauty, empowering her to feel more beautiful, sexy, visible, polished, less weary, whatever it is she desires. That's why I call this stage, the one you'll find at the very pinnacle of the PAP, optimization.

The optimization category includes BTX but also the other category of injectables, fillers. And I've also included some EBD treatments here. While the EBDs in the previous chapter were about stimulating the skin to regenerate, these EBDs are about erasing signs of damage and correcting skin, in particular treating red veins and pigmentation, but also smoothing surface texture and wrinkles.

I am seeing a slow but certain shift in how people view aesthetic treatments. In the industry there's a definite movement away from the humanoid look of the frozen forehead and Spock brows. We've come a long way from that old-fashioned male Harley Street cosmetic surgeon version of beautiful.

I am known for a look that's as pared back and as natural as possible. My approach is about being bespoke to each person's face, to celebrate their individuality. As you know, my focus is on the overall face, not on single wrinkles. The key to successful treatment is the blink impression, the impression your face first makes in a 'blink' of someone else's eye: shape, expression, skin tone and clarity. Used alone or along with injectables, EBDs can play a big part in that too.

What I want is for you to leave the clinic looking like you on a good day. Because there is no such thing as *anti*-ageing. We all age. What aesthetics allows you to do is become a version of yourself that feels more like you.

As I've said throughout the book, the work you have at this final layer of the PAP has its best results only when you've got your skin into great condition by doing the lower layers: in particular lifestyle (Chapter 3), skincare (Chapter 4) and facials (Chapter 6).

And I want to underline: this stage is in no way compulsory – some of the most beautiful faces I've seen have had no 'work' at all. This chapter is to let you know what can be done, the risks and benefits, so you can then make an informed and empowered decision about your own bespoke approach to positive ageing.

The new look 'tweakments'

Since BTX arrived 30 years ago, it's been a game-changer for the cosmetic market. Before BTX, the only options were surgery or fat transplant, both of which often gave a distinctive and unflattering aesthetic: the 'windswept' or 'tunnel' look.

Even the way BTX was first used, with frozen domed forehead and overly arched brows, looks outdated now. The same is true of fillers; their application has changed radically over time too. Whereas it used to be about filling out specific lines, it's now about enhancing the contours and proportions of the face. That said, there's still a lot of bad information and bad work out there. That is why I have had to put clients on BTX and filler detoxes when they come to me having overdone it (see page 229).

When I do injectables, I'm not looking to erase the signs of ageing - but to tweak them for a natural, subtle, fresher and firmer appearance. The aim, as with every stage of the PAP, is to enhance your features as opposed to looking like someone else's ideal of 'beautiful'.

Like most women I see in clinic, you will probably consider coming for treatment as a big step. The average time between my clients considering booking an appointment and actually coming in is 2 years. A 2015 study of 1,000 women by Ehlinger-Martin et al. saw that while 50% had considered injectable treatments, only 10% went ahead. If you've never had a treatment, you've likely got a lot of questions, including what might go wrong and how to get the best effect. I've included a general section to introduce BTX and fillers, but I think the best way to give you the information you need is by answering all the most common questions I am asked, day in day out, which I have done on pages 231–8.

I want to arm you with the facts so that you can better understand both the power and limitations of injectables, as well as the reasons why I believe things often go so wrong.

The point is, the tiniest of changes can transform your blink impression from one that's negative - perhaps angry, serious, worried or sad - to one that is energetic, healthy and positive. And your blink impression is how I judge the success of treatment.

Botulinum toxin (BTX)

This injectable treatment is both super-effective and considered very safe. BTX works by weakening the overactive facial muscles and so softening the wrinkles they cause. In the upper face in particular, the main contributing factor to the lines you see is repeated muscle movement, which leads to wear and tear, which then shows up as wrinkles. BTX slows down this whole process.

The most effective and dramatic results come from treating the vertical lines between the brows, often called the 11s, caused by frowning downwards. The next most effective place is the crows' feet, caused by smiling widely. Lifting up your brows is what causes the horizontal lines across your forehead. You can soften these lines but it takes skill and a light touch with the needle. You want to lose that permanent frown but you don't want to lose your expression.

Other good uses in the lower face - but they will depend on your face - are to lift the corners of the mouth, to smooth the chin, and to make the jawline and neck look firmer; although some people don't see any benefits from BTX in the lower face.

Botox™ has become something of a household name, but is actually just a brand name of the first botulinum type-A toxin to launch in the cosmetic market. In terms of growth, it is projected that Botox (the brand) will register nearly $8,000 million in revenue in 2023, up from $3,840 million in 2017. Along with Bocouture™ and Azzalure™ (also called Xeomin™ and Dysport™ respectively), these are the three main brands available in the UK market. Each practitioner will likely have their preference - but there is very little difference between them.

BTX has to be prescribed by a doctor, although it can be injected by anyone (not that you want it to be!). First approved by the FDA in 1989 for the treatment of strabismus, aka squint, it's been used for decades in hospital medicine. It's also used to treat incontinence (by being injected into the bladder), migraine and muscle stiffness. It has been used 'off licence' to treat wrinkles for 30 years; in the US it was officially approved for cosmetic use in 2002.

Very, very occasionally, it doesn't work. I have seen 3 cases in 15 years where the treatment doesn't have any effect, and it's not worth people having the treatment. There's a side-effect that's a little more common - I see up to 10 a year - where the effect wears off more quickly than expected, even after increasing the dose. I've found this can sometimes be solved by switching brands, although there's no research on this.

If you're worried about underwhelming or unwanted results, the key is the skill of your practitioner. It takes skill and experience to get the right amount of product in the right place. You do not want an unqualified practitioner with a production line of 20 clients per day, who injects in the same place in every face. You want someone who looks at the whole of your face, including while it's moving, before injecting, even if only treating one part, who does a follow-up and uses that information to tweak the next treatment in your programme.

The trend is now to use lower doses than before, because you really can have too much BTX. Especially as you age, too much can flatten brows, and it can make your face look shiny in parts and so emphasize crêpiness and a loss of firmness in other parts.

I am super-conservative about the age you start using BTX. I don't usually treat clients under 30, unless deep lines have already formed and are taking their toll psychologically. I do, however, advise starting before the lines have become etched in. You may be surprised to find that I usually reduce the dose used in the upper face with age. This is often to make sure, as the lower face ages, that the upper face doesn't look completely different or your expression too flat. In fact, I often stop treating the forehead completely in the 40s, depending on your facial structure and concerns. If it doesn't leave your eyes looking hooded or tired, you might still be able to get away with forehead BTX in light doses.

One of my favoured BTX techniques is sprinkles. This is the name for droplets placed superficially in the skin so they don't weaken all layers of a muscle. They soften lines while keeping movement.

As I'm known for this subtle approach, clients do come to me when they - or their practitioner - have overdone the work. I believe in injecting BTX dynamically, so lines may be softened but expressions aren't affected. And zooming out to see the whole impression of the face rather than looking at each wrinkle.

WHO IS IT FOR: Age 30+. Frown lines, wrinkles on the forehead, crows' feet. Some lower face benefits too, for example downturned mouth, clenched jaw, bumpy chin, visible neck bands.
TIME: 15 minutes (for a repeat treatment). First the skin is cleaned, then the injection points are marked up. The injections themselves take just a few minutes to perform. Injections do sting a little, but only at the moment they are made. The least number of injections is 3, probably the very most is 30.
DISCOMFORT: 1 out of 3.
DOWNTIME: You may have little bumps immediately afterwards, but these will settle within 15 minutes. The results take around 5 days to kick in, though they can occasionally take up to 2 weeks.
RESULTS: The results last between 2 and 6 months, depending on the dose and area treated. Treatment of crows' feet will typically last a maximum of 3 months, even at a very high dose, whereas treatment of frown lines can last 6 months.
PRICE: From £270. Clients usually attend clinic 3 to 4 times per year.

Hyaluronic acid (HA) fillers

We've met hyaluronic acid in previous chapters, as it's both naturally occurring in skin, a moisturizing skincare ingredient, and the key ingredient in skin booster treatments. Filler is simply HA made into a liquid gel implant that's injected deeper into your skin. This can be anywhere on the face, but most commonly lips, cheeks, temples, around the mouth, jawline and chin.

Fillers with a watery consistency are great for filling out surface fine lines and wrinkles, such as vertical lip lines and crows' feet at the sides of the eyes. Thicker, more viscous products are more appropriate for lifting and contouring the cheeks, chin and jawline.

After injection, there's an immediate, visible effect - what you see is what you get. Your skin forms a mesh around the HA, so it becomes part of the skin. There might be bumps at first, but from around 4 days in, you shouldn't be able to feel anything except an increased density in your skin, and certainly no edges to where you've been injected.

Then, over the next few months, sometimes years, the filler is reabsorbed into the body. Some older kinds of filler, for example Radiesse or Sculptra, plumped by stimulating more natural collagen production. This is a concept that hugely appeals to me, but I much prefer HA because it can be dissolved almost instantly by being injected with an enzyme, hyaluronase. That said, HA fillers do stimulate collagen to some extent too, which is why the effects can last longer than the actual product being in your skin.

As fillers are not prescription products, there's no meaningful regulation on either the product or the practitioner. In the US, products do need to be FDA approved, but in the UK they only need a CE mark for medical devices. And as I said, anyone can inject. So all the onus is on you to find the right practitioner and the right filler. I'd advise you to find someone who's properly qualified and whose work you've seen and *trust* (see page 239).

Serious complications such as allergy are rare, but it's still good to go to a practitioner who can dissolve the fillers if needed, as not all provide this service. There's also a small risk of delayed hypersensitivity, where the body rejects the foreign body and the client presents several months after treatment with puffiness or swelling in the treated area. This is treatable, but sometimes requires injection of steroids, which has to be done by a doctor. One more serious - but thankfully rare - complication is where a filler blocks or compresses a blood vessel. The highest risk area for this is around the nose, which is why, in our clinic, only doctors with surgical training treat this area.

More often, the clients I have seen in clinic who come to me to have fillers dissolved have had too much product placed incorrectly. This is most usually in their lips but also in the cheeks. Remember, you really want to look like *you* after a treatment, which means subtlety is key. I am a huge believer in using the smallest amount of product for maximum support and effect.

When using fillers, it all comes back to proportions. I never take features, for example the cheeks or lips, out of context of the whole face. And I always treat keeping in mind how the face moves, its expressions and looking at the face from all angles, rather than thinking of a static photo as the end result.

There is a very confusing array of different brands of filler, with new ones released all the time. In my clinic we use HA fillers almost 100% of the time for their consistent, predictable results. The main UK brands are Juvederm, Teoxane, Belotero and Restylane. And within each range there are different densities of gel, used for different areas.

WHO IS IT FOR: Age 35+. To replace the loss of volume in the face that leads to wrinkles and early signs of sagging. It can also be used very effectively for 'beautification', but proceed with caution (see page 229, BTX detox). I do use it on younger faces to give, for example, more defined cheeks or tweak a profile, but I only do this after a very detailed consultation and getting to know a client's motivations.

TIME: 30 minutes. First the skin is cleaned, then the injection points are marked up. I combine needle and cannula techniques, depending on what I'm trying to achieve. A cannula is a blunt needle and using one allows me to fan a product as I put it in, coating the skin and giving less risk of bruising. The injections themselves may take from 5 to 45 minutes to perform, depending on how many.

DISCOMFORT: 1 to 2 out of 3. Most fillers are pre-mixed with anaesthetic so they sting a little less than BTX. I try to do as few injections as possible, as I want to avoid breaking the skin more than strictly necessary. Although you will feel the needle when it very first goes in, the feeling quickly becomes more of a dull ache or pressure - and in any case it only lasts a few seconds.

DOWNTIME: You might feel a little tender and puffy in the area - but only you will notice - for up to 4 or 5 days.

RESULTS: The results are visible immediately. Fillers will last from around 3 months to 18 months. The consistency of the filler will affect how long it lasts, as will the area used. Tear trough injections for under-eyes (see page 226) can last the longest, up to several years.

PRICE: From £300 (at my clinic) per syringe. Clients usually have from 1 to 4 syringes, and typically attend the clinic once per year.

CASE STUDY

A natural look

Jane, 33, is a psychologist who spends a lot of her time working with clients. She came to see me because she noticed that the lines on her forehead were getting deeper and more etched, even though she's only in her early 30s. I noticed she was frowning all the time, even as she spoke to me. Even Jane's resting face was beginning to look cross and intense, the opposite of the approachable and friendly impression she wanted to make at work. And even, a lot of the time, the opposite of how she was feeling. She hadn't realized she was frowning so much.

Because Jane needs to empathize with people, and an important part of that is mirroring the other person's expression, she really needed to retain movement in her face.

It's a very common misconception that if you treat the frown you won't be able to lift your eyebrows. In fact, it's a separate group of muscles that lift the eyebrows and cause horizontal frown lines to those that bring the brows together and cause vertical frown lines. Jane had come to me because she wanted to frown less, but also because she heard that my approach to BTX is to be targeted and minimal. In the first appointment, I also re-evaluated and scaled down her skincare regime.

Jane had her first two BTX treatments 4 months apart. I didn't completely block the whole width of the frown, rather I concentrated on softening the 11s by treating the muscle at the top of her nose. She could still move her forehead and frown and express her emotion, but not with the same intensity. Over time, as she got used to not having the ability to frown downwards, she ended up training herself out of that mannerism. Now, the lines haven't come back. She can have less BTX and she has it only twice a year.

Blink impression tweaks

Sad?

Downward turned corners of the mouth

Applying BTX to the muscle that is pulling the corners of the lips down can give a very subtle lift. It might be only millimetres, but it works. The added bonus of this is that when you are talking, laughing or eating, the whole mouth area can appear firmer.

Deep frown furrows

BTX reduces the movement of the muscles that make you frown, which in itself lightens your look. Also, as you frown, the constant contraction actually stimulates collagenase, the enzyme that breaks collagen down. So, during the time the BTX is active, the actual wrinkles have time to repair and the skin has time to heal - another benefit of weakening that movement.

Tired?

Droopy eyelids, dark circles

Carefully placed BTX can give the tail of the brow a tiny lift, just 2-3mm, but enough to make the whole eye area feel more open and look more rested. There's a fat pad that sits on the orbit bone, the circular bone you can feel underneath the eye. It often flattens with age, making dark circles more prominent. You can treat dark circles with what's called 'tear trough filler'. This involves injecting droplets of filler gel directly on to the orbit bone. The injections pad out the under-eye, so reducing the appearance of the circles.

Old?

A changing face shape

At 25 years old, your face has full temples, high cheeks and a firm jawline. This is called the triangle of youth, with the wider part at the top. As you age this shape reverses; the temples hollow out, the beautiful curve of the cheek flattens, and you may develop jowls. Where you sit in this process is a big factor in the blink impression. You can change this impression using fillers to add volume and define.

CASE STUDY

Treating jowls with fillers

Roberta, 53, came to me saying she had begun to dislike catching sight of herself in the mirror. She said that she had become very self-conscious about her jowls in particular.

Part of the reason Roberta notices her jowls is that she has what's called a short chin. That is, the distance between her lower lip and chin is relatively small. There is considered to be an 'ideal' in lower face proportions. And it is that the measurement between the nose and mouth should ideally be half the measurement between the mouth and chin. But as we age, the chin gets shorter and wider. The shorter the chin, the more likely that the beginning of jowling – that we all get – will be noticeable.

We also discussed the impact of teeth grinding on her facial shape – her lower face had widened, giving a squareness. She also has noticeable dark circles under her eyes, although she's not as bothered by them as by her jowls. When I mentioned them, she laughed and said she'd got used to looking tired.

The first step, following the principles of the PAP, was to get Roberta's skin into better condition with skincare and facials. She also had a regenerative treatment, ultrasound, to help with firming and tightening the skin.

Roberta was a good candidate for fillers. I did tell her that she'd need an amount that was going towards the most I'd inject. The first place I injected fillers was into her chin, to the sides and also in the front, so that it projected more. Elongating the chin in this way is a small tweak that makes the jawline look more defined. It subtly changes the angles of the face, so the face looks less boxy and masculine, more v-shaped. And because it goes against how we age, it gives the face a slightly younger look, too.

Secondly, I worked on the mid-face, contouring Roberta's cheeks and again bringing back the v-shape of her younger face. I injected along the cheekbone and into the apples of the cheek, mostly at a deep level. This wasn't to give her new cheekbones but to replace the fat that Roberta had lost over time. This fat loss is what causes nose to mouth lines (nasolabial folds) and the beginning of jowling. The desired effect is to subtly enhance contours, as if you're wearing blusher.

I also injected BTX into Roberta's masseters, the jaw muscles. This was to ease the grinding and slightly reduce the width of her lower jaw, making her cheeks look more lifted, and distracting from the loss of elasticity in her jaw area.

Finally, Roberta had a few drops of tear trough fillers, placed precisely on the orbit bone of her eye socket, to deal with her dark circles. Filler can't treat bulging eye bags and it can't take away the darkness, but it can make dark under-eyes look less pronounced by changing the way the light bounces off them.

Admittedly, Roberta had a largish budget. She spent close to £1,600 on fillers and BTX alone. And this is probably close to the maximum amount I'd inject. But she is delighted with the results and says it has left her feeling much more cheerful and confident. She says it's better than spending the money on a holiday.

BTX DETOX

Sadly, I've seen this become an increasingly popular and necessary treatment option after people have had too much BTX for too long. It's all too easy to get caught up in the thrill of being able to make small but dramatic changes. I've found that stopping treatment, then starting fresh, can work wonders, give someone a physical and psychological reset, even if they're resistant at first.

You'll need to go cold turkey for 4 months for BTX, and up to a year for fillers. It allows me to really see your face, your blink impression, your contours. You may get your wrinkles back, or some of them. Your face will likely feel saggier and more lined to you than it looks to other people.

When I train new doctors I always stress that a big part of our job is to 'hold the reins' and if this means stopping treatment, so be it. But this will also require a lengthy initial consultation and detailed assessments, with an annual treatment plan where regular review is key. A detox allows you to go back to the PAP and decide an annual plan that will get you the results you want, within your budget. That usually ends up being way smaller doses than before.

CASE STUDY

A BTX detox

When I first met Jo, 47, she'd had over 10 years of BTX and fillers, starting in her mid-30s. She came to me asking for more. After talking about what she really wanted to achieve and discussing how this treatment was making her feel, she admitted that she didn't feel good, that her face didn't look quite right. She confessed that she'd begun to feel she didn't look like herself.

There is a same-y look that can happen if you keep having treatment, year in year out. It flattens your face and knocks out any expression at all. That's especially true if the treatment has been tailored for the person to look good while their face is static, rather than being designed around their expressions while their face is moving or they are talking. When injectables have been overdone, you can look smooth and perfect in pictures but quite alien as your face moves. At the same time, Jo hated her wrinkles and was scared to let them come back.

Jo's first consultation was in January. When she came in, she was wearing a lot of make-up to disguise the redness of her skin. She told me her skin often flared up while she was stressed and got worse in the winter, particularly around Christmas. She often got spots before her period, too. Jo has two small children, runs her own business, and is a self-confessed exercise junkie. She runs so she can keep her weight down and eat what she likes. Even her vigorous exercise schedule was stressful. She was doing boxing, weight training, running (including marathon length runs), and lots and lots of intense ashtanga yoga.

My first advice to Jo was for her to find time and space to de-stress. That included doing exercise with less impact and more regenerative qualities, such as finding a softer form of yoga than ashtanga.

Jo was open to a nutritional approach, to address redness and breakouts. She followed a 12-week programme devised by our nutritional therapist. In particular she was advised to watch her sugar intake.

Like Jo's fast-paced life, she was using intense skincare too, full of active ingredients. But you can have too much of a good thing when it comes to skincare. One reason for the redness of her skin was that her barrier needed supporting. I advised her to cut down her products (see page 152 for a programme for redness) and she was also prescribed some topical medication by our dermatologist.

To Jo's dismay, I put her on a BTX detox for 4 months, to wait for it to wear off. I then put a light dose of BTX into her frown and the tails of her brows for a slight lift, plus a tweak to the side of her mouth to take away the little down-turning there. And that was it.

The fillers took longer to wear off, around a year. Once that had happened, I could reassess her face, and we both agreed she didn't need nearly as much, and only in her cheeks. She had Profhilo for a hydration boost and to improve the texture of her skin, especially in her neck as it looked more crêpey than her face.

As Jo saw her skin change and start to look healthy, she could see the benefit of not having every line filled. Now she loves the fact that she can go to the school gate wearing no make-up if she wants to, that she has that choice. She also says her make-up goes on a lot better, too.

Fears I hear about injectables

You say: 'I don't want to be putting chemicals and foreign bodies into my skin'

BTX is a toxin, that is true, but in cosmetic medicine we use a purified and heavily diluted form. The dosages are a fraction of what is used in hospital medicine. For example, a 2-year-old with cerebral palsy might receive a 2,000-unit dose to stop muscle contraction and so allow her to walk. But a typical cosmetic dose can start at 6 units. The systemic effects of the drug have been well studied at much higher doses and it is still considered very safe.

The product is sold to doctors as a powder in the bottom of a vial, which the doctor then dilutes and activates for injection using saline. The dosage is already measured out in the vials.

The botulinum toxin is quickly metabolized, so doesn't hang around in the body very long - some studies suggest just hours. It leaves behind the relaxed muscles that, in the right hands, can make such a difference to the look of the face.

When it comes to fillers, HA is a naturally occurring substance that your body produces, uses and replenishes daily. Around 50% of your body's HA is found in skin, but it's also an important component of the cartilage that sits between muscle layers. In the body, it acts as a hydrator, lubricator for your joints, and antioxidant. Over a period of months, the HA in fillers is reabsorbed into the body.

You say: 'I'm scared of pain/needles'

Being nervous about needles is pretty common. And it's logical: who would want a needle put into them? The problem is, if you feel fear, that psychological component can lead to tense muscles - and that can make the first time more painful.

I want to reassure you; it's normal to feel some hesitation. But I also want to reassure you that the needles used are absolutely tiny. Even people who've baulked at the idea of needles at first will often come back for their second treatment feeling excited, as they know how good they'll feel afterwards.

There are lots of techniques and tricks that can help distract you from what the practitioner is doing. Most fillers are now pre-mixed with anaesthetic, which means that additional anaesthetic creams or injections are usually not required. Though there are some more sensitive areas - the skin above your upper lip, for example - where a topical anaesthetic cream is usually enough. You might also be offered ice to numb the skin, or a little vibrating T-bar to hold, to draw your senses away from what the practitioner is doing.

There is also distraction: some clients prefer to chat through a procedure, others do better by being in their zone, using breathing techniques or listening to music. Some patients have found hypnosis useful before they have come into clinic.

My advice is to be open about how you feel about injections with your practitioner before you get into the chair. It's also a good idea to book your appointment according to your menstrual cycle. People often find that their skin is more sensitive just before their period.

You say: 'Others will notice the difference/I won't look like me'
This is all down to the skill of the practitioner. The aim is to look like the best version of you - or even you after a holiday. It is a failure on their part if you do not feel this way after treatment, and you should always say to your practitioner if you aren't happy with the results. This doesn't happen very often, as I find that when you get the consultation right - with transparency about costs - then you should get the right result. But your practitioner should always be prepared to talk to you and give you a follow-up.

To find a practitioner, follow the instructions on page 239. Then, at your initial consultation, make sure you discuss your motivation for having treatment now, and your long-term goals too. Ask the practitioner: are there alternatives to injectables? Is there a more holistic skincare approach? Do you need them now or can you wait? Is the practitioner going to create you a treatment plan of what is best to have and when? Have you discussed your budget for this, in time as well as money? Transparency regarding prices is important. And I'd always recommend a slowly, slowly, step-by-step approach, over months rather than weeks.

Finally, if you have a consultation and aren't entirely convinced, walk away and look for someone else. It is entirely your decision. You have to be happy.

You say: 'I'm concerned about cost'

This will depend on the practitioner's qualifications and level of experience (alongside the location and the facilities). Take these points into consideration when weighing up your options:

- Don't be led by price. To an extent, yes, you have your budget, as with all areas of life. But, if you can, try not to be swayed by bargains and discounts. I realize this may be easier said than done.
- Think about the cost per use! Fillers (from £300 per syringe) can last 6 to 18 months, and BTX (from £270) can last 2 to 6 months. So they are arguably better value in cost-per-use terms than the handbag or shoes you might splurge on. (But then again, I'm biased.)
- Make sure your practitioner helps you to prioritize treatments. It is part of our job to help you to get clear about your goals, priorities, timeline and best bang for buck.

BTX: I recommend repeating before the effects have completely worn off, as there is a cumulative effect. After a few treatments they will start to last longer, as there will be a time-lag between muscle movement returning and wrinkles reappearing because skin has improved. The upside? A more natural result, as you'll need smaller and smaller doses.

FILLERS: Every face is different and a lot depends on lifestyle, such as diet, exercise, sleep. But 1 to 2 syringes each year in your 30s is usually a good preventative/maintenance strategy. An initial 'kick-start' in your

40s might involve 3 to 4 syringes but then an annual maintenance of 1 to 2 syringes. From your 50s onwards, 2 syringes can still make a big difference. Then again, I can use 8 syringes and it still looks natural, just softter and fresher. Remember: 5 syringes is just a teaspoon, so we're not talking large volumes.

You say: 'I'm scared something's going to go horribly wrong'

BTX and fillers are what I have done, day in, day out, for the past 15 years. I am very comfortable with their risk and benefit profile. Of course, every treatment has its risks: make sure you have been guided through a thorough and informed consent process with your practitioner. Every one of your concerns is valid until you have received adequate reassurance! Do your research and go to a reputable clinic (see page 239). Be open to visiting more frequently at the start of your programme to get best results, rather than having all your treatment, all at once.

Genuine BTX allergy is extremely rare and usually presents with nausea and general malaise, which subsides after a few days. The side-effects of BTX are possible bruising or headaches, but these are rare, mild, and usually just on the day of treatment. Complications are not common and are usually cosmetic. Be careful not to apply pressure to the area in the days following treatment (to avoid the product moving and weakening muscles your practitioner was not intending to weaken).

BTX weakens muscles - this is how it works - so if the dose is wrong it is possible to cause droopy eyelids. This can happen when the practitioner treats the columns of forehead muscles that lift the brows up and that cause horizontal forehead lines, but these muscles become overwhelmed. This can lead to the 'BTX droop' or ptosis (this means heavy lids). This is always temporary, should ease on its own in a few weeks and can sometimes be improved with further injections.

Badly done BTX can also lead to Spock eyes, that startled look and unnaturally shaped raised brow. You do not have to live with this, as it's super-simple to correct. Just ask for a follow-up appointment! The same goes for the 'comma lines' that sometimes appear just above the tail of your brows after treatment. They are easily fixed with a couple of additional drops of BTX.

FILLERS: There is a higher rate of complications with fillers but the huge benefit is that - unlike BTX - HA fillers are reversible. Again, the most common problem here is a poor cosmetic result, a 'paint by numbers' approach, with new cheeks, jawline and lips being applied to a face without a thorough assessment and out of context to the full face proportions and 'blink impression'.

The other common concern that I hear is the risk of the filler moving after being injected - 'migration'. This is not common, but it does happen. Usually it's barely noticeable, if at all. It won't move far, and if HA fillers have been used it is correctable. Product choice and technique are very important here. Again, practitioner experience is key.

And remember, if you are not happy, go back to your practitioner! This is always best, as they know the exact details of the treatment.

You say: 'I'm worried about bruising and swelling' OR 'How long is the recovery time?'

For most people, there is very little bruising or swelling after injectables, but there is no 100% guarantee. After you have BTX, it takes 15 minutes for the bumps where you've been injected to go down. You will need to refrain from exercise for 24 hours, and no facial massage or pressure to the area treated for 1 week.

There is usually just a little redness where you've had fillers, and you might be slightly puffy. It's best not to put make-up on for 12 hours, so schedule for a time when you have no important meetings for the rest of the day. Same as BTX, no massage for 1 week.

- To avoid bruising, avoid painkillers and alcohol in the days preceding treatment. Even one glass of wine the night before can make a difference. Also avoid omega-3 fish oils, vitamin E and ginger, as they increase the risk of bruising.
- Taking arnica tablets, a high dose, for 1 week beforehand can help too.
- Apply vitamin K cream after the treatment. This doesn't prevent bruising like arnica does, but will break down the purple colour of a bruise much faster.
- Dermablend, an effective concealing make-up, is quite brilliant!

You say: 'I am worried about the long-term effects. If I stop having treatments, will the ageing process be accelerated?!'
Quick answer: No! If you've heard that BTX is preventative, it's not just hype. For as long as BTX is active, you are actually slowing down the ageing process by reducing wear and tear. I often look back on pictures with clients who had deep furrows – most often the 11s or vertical lines – 10 years before, that have been completely erased over time with gentle but regular treatments.

And as for deciding to stop, if you do there will be no abrupt decline, especially if you have been following a programme including skincare, etc. A lot of my clients stop and start because of pregnancy and breastfeeding. And they find that even with the impact of exhaustion, hormones and weight changes, the work they've had previously holds them in good stead and makes any work they have after stopping breastfeeding take effect quickly and easily.

You say: 'My partner is completely against treatments' OR 'My work colleagues would frown on me having treatments' OR 'Absolutely no one can know I am doing this!'
This is the most personal 'fear' I hear from clients. And when it comes to fear of being judged by colleagues, I get it. I have clients who work for non-profit organizations, or have seen friends lose their jobs, and

who struggle with the guilt or perceive having treatment as being insensitive. If this sounds like you, I'd like to direct you back to my earlier chapter covering mindset (see page 38), so you can explore your own conflict and feelings, if you haven't already.

When women tell me their partners won't be OK with them having treatment, it makes me quite emotional! The two most common reasons they state are, first, that their partner would be scared of something not going well, which is, as you know, a very low risk. And second, the cost. But it is YOUR FACE, YOUR CHOICE. It is OK to want to feel like the best version of you. And it is no one else's business what you do with your body.

On the wider - how will society judge me? - scale of things, this is one of the reasons I am writing this book. For too long 'ageing' has been used against women as something they should be ashamed of, or as a tool to market more expensive - and ineffective - products towards. I'm a huge believer in educating yourself on what you are doing in order to be sure it is right for you. There is no shame in this.

And finally, if you really don't want anyone to know, be honest with your practitioner about what aesthetic outcome you want. It is very easy to achieve a natural look these days.

FILLER TRENDS

- **Lips:** As I'm sure you know by now, I don't like the over-plumped look. So can lip filler ever look OK? Yes! Lips deflate with age, just like the rest of your face. Restoring plumpness here is an important part of facial rejuvenation. It is absolutely possible to do this without distorting shape - with the appropriate technique and product.

- **Noses:** Some of the results I've seen of HA fillers being used for non-surgical rhinoplasty have astounded me. Fillers can give incredible results, but without the risks, downtime and permanence of surgery. However, the (small) risks of hitting a blood vessel and blocking blood flow to the area are higher when injecting this area, so in our clinic only doctors with surgical training perform this treatment.
- **Jawline and chin:** the latest 'buzz' area. Better definition at the angle of the jaw and very slight enhancements to the point of your chin can do wonders for the early signs of sag.

HOW TO FIND A GOOD INJECTABLE PRACTITIONER

You might be surprised to know that while BTX has to be prescribed by a doctor, nurse prescriber or dentist, fillers do not. They can be bought and injected by anyone in the UK. However, you need to have been accepted on to an accredited course to get insurance. But there are a lot of people injecting without insurance. So, when you are researching clinic websites, do check the practitioner's level of qualifications. I'd recommend injectables are done by a doctor, dentist or nurse, because of their clinical training and knowledge of anatomy.

Next, the practitioner must have the right level of experience. How many years have they been doing non-surgical treatments? How many aesthetic clients do they see each week (i.e. is it a sideline to their day job)? Make sure they belong to a relevant regulatory body. These are: BCAM (British College of Aesthetic Medicine); BACN (British Association of Cosmetic Nurses);

CQC (Care Quality Commission); GDC (General Dental Council).

When you go for your consultation, ask to see pictures of clients, in particular those like you or those who are having a similar treatment plan. Look around the waiting room at the clients and look at the faces of the staff.

Finally, when you have your consultation, be clear about the look you're going for. Make sure that what they say is a good outcome for you, is what you want.

Optimizing skin

I described EBDs in the last chapter in terms of *regeneration*, in that they can firm skin by stimulating new collagen and elastin production. In this chapter, I've included EBDs that have more of a corrective, optimizing effect. There are so many devices, but I have focused on the two categories of treatment most useful and popular in the clinic: fractional lasers for skin resurfacing and the EBDs (lasers and IPL) that target uneven skin tone: brown spots and burst vessels.

Fractional lasers

These devices target and heat water in the skin, causing controlled tissue injury that triggers skin resurfacing (improving texture and evening out skin tone) as well as some new collagen and elastin production in the dermis. As these lasers have a stronger effect on the epidermis than the EBDs in the previous chapter, they often each result in more downtime, too.

Earlier versions of this used the old style of laser that completely removed the epidermal layer, damaging it so it scabbed over, allowing a new face of fresher, unblemished skin to grow back. Those lasers are less popular now, mainly because the downtime is so long. Also, they had a high risk of complications in the healing period, including infection as you're effectively left with an open wound. After the procedure, skin is left highly sensitized for months, which carries an increased risk of pigmentation too.

Fractional lasers are the new generation. Invented in the Noughties, these are now much more popular than the old-school technique of complete resurfacing. They're called fractional because only a 'fraction' of skin is treated with each pass - through multiple, microscopically small columns. Each stamp with the laser head causes a grid of tiny channels of burnt skin. The surrounding skin then gets to work healing these wounds, creating lots more collagen and elastin, as well as new blood vessels.

When thinking about brands in this area, Fraxel is like the Hoover of treatments, as it's by far the most well-known, but actually there are many different devices available. They will differ by which wavelength they fire at, as well as by how much damage they do the epidermis.

An ablative laser (e.g. Fraxel Repair or Lumenis Fx) will remove the epidermal layer of each tiny micro-channel it creates. Downtime will be greater (around 1 week), but usually only a single treatment is required, with maintenance every 1 to 2 years. Good for fine wrinkles (e.g. the under-eye area) and pigmentation.

A 'non-ablative' laser (e.g. ICON1540) causes much less damage to the epidermis, while still triggering plenty of remodelling in the deeper layers. A course is required, but downtime is far more manageable, usually just a few days of mild swelling and possibly flaking.

WHO IS IT FOR: Age 45+. To 'resurface' - improve texture, tone and wrinkles. People often start using this laser to treat lip lines or crêpey under-eye areas, then like the effects so much that they progress to full face. Also good for addressing acne scarring.

TIME: 1 hour including anaesthetic cream.
DISCOMFORT: 2 out of 3. It does require anaesthetic cream and it will burn afterwards for 45 minutes to an hour.
DOWNTIME: Depending on the strength of the laser used and the area covered, 12 hours to 1 week. You may be red, and have puffiness, dryness and flaking.
RESULTS: You start seeing results at 4 to 6 weeks. It's a fantastic treatment as part of a long-term programme. Repeat the course every 2 years.
PRICE: £700+.

Vascular lasers and IPL

These devices also generate high-energy beams of light, pushed into the face via a handpiece. To treat redness, the machine will target the red haemoglobin found in blood cells and vessels. To treat brown spots, the machine will target the melanin.

Different machines will specialize in different wavelengths to target particular issues. Different intensities for different indications will also affect how much recovery time you will need.

IPL looks and acts like a laser but does not qualify as a 'true' laser, as the handpiece delivers multiple wavelengths of light, i.e. multiple targets, simultaneously. IPL is a very useful machine; with minimal recovery time, it's the accepted first-line treatment for pigmentation, redness, acne, early textural complexion changes and even hair removal (it targets the brown or melanin in hair too).

WHO IS IT FOR: Age 30+. IPL is often the first treatment people have for most pigmentation and/or redness. Sometimes a vascular laser (e.g. Excel V or V-Beam) is required for resistant vessels around the nose or more advanced rosacea.
TIME: 15 to 45 minutes.
DISCOMFORT: 2 out of 3. Uncomfortable but usually just for the split second the device fires.

DOWNTIME: Depends on the strength of the treatment, i.e. extent of red/brown being treated. Red: from flushing for an hour or so, to bruising and puffiness that can last up to a week. Brown: will darken almost immediately - and take up to 1 week to lighten.
RESULTS: Can be immediate for redness - especially dramatic around the nose, where a single treatment can last for 6 months or more. Many of my clients will return for a single IPL maintenance treatment after an initial course.
PRICE: From £200. An initial course of 3 treatments, 1 month apart, is usually recommended.

PDO Thread lifts

These are useful when EBDs are no longer giving enough of a tightening result and more fillers will distort, not lift. They have a place when clients need a lift but are not interested in surgery.

The practitioner inserts fine surgical-grade 'barbed' threads from the mouth and chin area up to the hairline, effectively pulling the skin upwards, lifting the face. They are sutures, the same things surgeons use for stitches, but they have tiny bumps or barbs along the length to keep them in place. They can be placed from the temple to the jawline to smooth very early jowls. Or from the temple to the brow for a brow lift, or from the temple to the nasolabial fold for a mid-cheek lift.

There are many different designs and brands of threads: I prefer the ones with barbs, as I've seen them achieve faster, more consistent results. But every practitioner will have their preference.

The procedure involves no cutting or stitching, just a fine cannula (blunt needle) insertion to guide the sutures. The sutures then break down over approximately 6 months. But the reaction of the tissues around the thread tends to hold results for up to 18 months. We often recommend a few additional threads for the jawline at around 9 months.

WHO IS IT FOR: Age 45+. It's for the first signs of sagging.
TIME: 45 minutes.
DISCOMFORT: 1 to 2 out of 3.
DOWNTIME: Up to 1 week of puffiness, swelling and/or bruising. And it will feel very tight for 2 to 3 days after the procedure, especially when talking or eating.
RESULTS: Results are subtle - and usually last around 12 to 18 months for the lower face, 6 months for brow lifts. It's so important to be very clear regarding expectations, so do discuss it with your practitioner in detail. Even though results are subtle, they can make a big difference, especially when combined with injectables and EBDs for maintenance. But all this isn't cheap. It might be a better use of your time and money to consider surgery.
PRICE: It's a one-off treatment but you can have a booster of fewer threads. £2,000 for 15 threads (full-face treatment).

FIXES FOR TIRED EYES

You inherit a tendency to dark shadows under the eyes, and a lot of women are pretty conscious about this. Treatment for this will depend on what's causing it, and there is often more than one issue going on. Lifestyle changes and skincare can help (see page 36) but these treatments are the next level.

1. Dark circles

If your dark circles are a brown colour, they're likely due to pigmentation. If you have tried skincare (see page 157) and it hasn't worked, this can be treated with peeling (see page 192) or intensive mesotherapy (see page 205; 6 treatments, done every 2 weeks for 12 weeks, £600 for the course).

Discoloration that's more of a purple colour is likely to be due to leaking blood vessels. Lasers and IPL can work here, but be sure to see a skilled practitioner who's experienced in treating this delicate area.

Another option is tear trough filler (explained on page 226), a tiny amount of filler injected under the eye to lift the hollowing that can often worsen the appearance of dark circles.

2. Eye bags

These are, for the most part, genetic and worsen as you age. Sometimes they can be indirectly improved by addressing volume loss in the cheek and tear trough area using fillers. But this is disguising the issue rather than treating it. See point 4 below for more.

3. Fine lines

A lot of my clients come in after having noticed lines around their eyes - and on their forehead - from squinting at a screen. BTX is a very effective treatment for crows' feet (see page 219). And there are skin boosters that work for this area: Redensity 1 and Sunekos. Another option is mesotherapy, which is tiny, shallow injections of vitamins (see page 205).

Deeper lines, crows' feet that can still be seen at rest, or that have started to work their way down the cheek, respond well to Tixel (see page 214) or resurfacing lasers. There is downtime - some swelling, tiny scabs and flaking - for up to a week with these procedures, and sometimes they need to be repeated for best results.

4. Crêpey skin and/or loss of elasticity

Radio-frequency needling, such as Morpheus 8, can be effective here. However, for upper lids I often find myself encouraging clients to consider a consultation with an oculoplastic surgeon for blepharoplasty (a type of surgery that repairs droopy eyelids and may involve removing excess skin, muscle and fat). Because you'll only see minimal improvement with non-surgical treatments, and the results will last 1 to 2 years at the most. Blepharoplasty is a relatively straightforward procedure that can be performed under local anaesthetic.

TARGETED TREATMENTS

NECK: This is a tricky area to treat and one where *prevention* is key. That means applying sunscreen and using your active skincare all the way down over the chest. Facials and skin-tightening treatments such as radiofrequency and ultrasound work here, as do needling, skin boosters and PRP. If the issue is down to over-activation of the neck muscle (the platysma), BTX may work here too.

Finally, there's Aqualyx (or Kybella in the US), which I haven't mentioned before. It's a fat-busting injection, good for reducing double chins. The active ingredient is deoxycholic acid, a naturally occurring molecule in the body that destroys fat cells. The procedure involves injections under the chin, which can be painful and usually cause bruising and a lot of swelling that can take up to a week to settle. But once destroyed, these cells can no longer store or accumulate fat, so results are permanent.

Price: From £600. A repeat treatment at 6 weeks may be required.

CHEST: The same applies as for the neck (see above) but surface texture is more of an issue here too. For pigmentation and redness, use IPL or a laser. For wrinkles or crêpiness, try medical needling (see page 203) or skin boosters (see page 208).

Price: From £240 for a single treatment of IPL or needling, from £390 for skin boosters.

LASER HAIR REMOVAL: You may find you get more hair as you age and plucking or waxing may be a trigger for post-inflammatory pigmentation. This treatment is both safe and effective. The laser works best when it can easily target the hair because there is greatest contrast between dark hair on pale skin. Sometimes touch-up annual maintenance sessions are required after completing a course.

Price: From £35 for a single treatment. Courses of 6–8 treatments are required. The ideal treatment interval varies depending on which area is being treated.

FAT-FREEZING: Cryolipolysis has turned out to be a big advance in non-surgical body contouring. The most common areas we treat in the clinic are the lower and upper abs and flanks. It can also be used under the chin. It's a very popular, non-invasive treatment for stubborn fat pockets. We use CoolSculpting® - a procedure that delivers precisely controlled cooling to target the fat cells underneath the skin. Treated fat cells are crystallized (frozen), effectively destroyed over the 30-minute treatment time. Then over several weeks your body naturally eliminates these dead cells. I'm a huge fan of its results. But I'm also a huge fan of exercise, for all its myriad benefits, both inside and out. That doesn't mean there isn't a place for this treatment, and I've seen it be very helpful post-childbirth and post-menopause. However, you do need to know it's not going to change your life and it cannot replace good food and exercise.

Price: From £600.

SKIN TAGS: These are very common, and can get more common with age. But they are also very easy to remove using radiosurgery. In a 10-minute session, up to 20 can be treated.

Price: From £150.

As you now know, BTX is far from being the only tool in the aesthetic medicine chest, although it's probably the most famous. By now, you also know all the levels of the PAP. In the next and final chapter, I'm going to help you work out how to build your own personal PAP.

COSMETIC SURGERY

Only a small percentage of my clients end up choosing surgery these days. This is largely because the advances in non-surgical procedures have reduced the need for it, and clients are becoming less comfortable with permanent changes. However, blepharoplasty, rhinoplasty, face, neck and brow-lifts are still common, very safe and can really improve problem areas.

Deciding on these sorts of procedures is very personal, and I always make sure my clients take time to consider both their mental and physical concerns. The cost can vary from £2,000 to £20,000, and recovery time can be several weeks, so I suggest only looking into this if you have completed the PAP and have a problem area that is still making you unhappy. A combined surgical and non-surgical approach can work really well. Typically my clients who decide to have 'lifting' surgery are 50+, but remember, age is just a number!

CHAPTER ROUND-UP

- What is your blink impression? How has it changed? What would you like it to be?
- Take your time to find a practitioner you like and trust: you should be on the same page in terms of cost, techniques and aesthetic outcome.
- BTX is a safe treatment.
- Never be ashamed about having treatments. YOUR FACE, YOUR CHOICE.

Chapter Nine

Making your plan

When I started out as an aesthetic doctor, my focus was on BTX and fillers, as I used to think that was the best way to get real results. But over the years, I've increasingly seen how vital lifestyle is to positive ageing. Having closely examined the skin of so many women over so many years, I've seen how reducing stress, eating well, exercising and getting in control of your hormones can transform skin better than any treatment in my arsenal.

Lifestyle medicine is now my personal passion, with its power to slow and even reverse the processes that happen as we age.

From the thousands of conversations I've had in clinic, I've seen how big a part mindset plays in the way you present to the world and approach the ageing process, too.

I've also seen what good skincare and maintenance can do to the function of your skin, and to the rate at which it slows the 5 signs of ageing. During my working life, companies have launched so many good technologies that really do restore skin and transform how it functions. There's so much expert information and so many incredible treatments that don't involve needles, so BTX and fillers have ended up being the cherry on top of what I offer in clinic, not the main course at all.

In this book, I've translated my 15 years of experience into an easy-to-follow programme: the Positive Ageing Pyramid. The PAP is a method for glowing skin at any age, and feeling good about it.

That's why I've given you the knowledge of how your skin works, and how it interacts with all the bewildering array of treatment options out there. Whatever you have decided, however high it suits you to climb up the pyramid, my goal has been to demystify the ageing process.

This last chapter is all about guiding you to design your own PAP – and set your priorities. I know you're probably short of time, and most of us don't have the money to do everything. Social events, family, financial and work pressures will always push and pull. None of us have enough time. It will help you to be clear about your priorities. And I hope the questions I'm about to ask will help you decide what they are.

Your annual plan

I suggest you create your PAP as an annual plan, with daily and weekly priorities. The great thing about planning ahead is that, once you've made the decisions, you don't have to think about them again or spend any unexpected funds. Appearance might be important to make you feel good, but so is making sure that it takes up as little headspace as possible.

With this in mind, setting strong foundations by working on *feeling* beautiful and establishing good lifestyle habits – what I call free cosmetic medicine! – are the first steps. And then it's all about educated decisions, based on realistic, clearly defined expectations and always in tune with your budget – both time and money.

Fortunately, there is no longer a one-fits-all idea of beauty. You can use this book to help you to look your best at any age. But ultimately, do whatever it takes to enjoy being you.

What to remember

Follow these principles while you're building your annual plan. Start by looking back at the notes you wrote as you read the book, what resonated with you, the parts you underlined. Now pick 3 to 5 changes to start you off. In my experience, fewer is best. It will be the handful of things that you jotted down because they are most compelling that will make the difference. For example, I would like to: do daily breathing exercises, focus on eating more fibre for my gut, work out my 5 skincare basics and start using them.

Then, when those are set in stone in your life, you can add to them if there are other things you want to address. But I often find that once people have started to tackle their core concerns, their list of 'things to change' dramatically reduces as they become more confident.

Building your PAP toolkit

Here are some prompts to help you reflect on the notes you have made, or thoughts you've had while reading. Scribble/circle - jot it down here and take your time to mull it over.

Mindset

Look in the mirror. What do you see? List 3 things you like, 3 things you don't like about your face.

....

....

....

....

....

If you could change one thing, what would it be?

....

Fill in this sentence:

....
will be better/happen once I fix this.

Now ask yourself: might you be expecting too much from aesthetic treatments? What other steps could you take right now? What's stopping you?

See Chapter 2 for more on how to get your mindset working for you.

Lifestyle medicine

Which lifestyle area are you going to start with? I've put some basic suggestions under each heading, but there are plenty more in Chapter 3, as you know!

Stress

[ ] Breathing better
[ ] Sleeping better
[ ] Exercise

Nutrition

[ ] Cutting down on sugar and/or alcohol
[ ] Cooking a diverse veg-filled diet; eating the rainbow
[ ] Supplements

Hormones

[ ] Cutting stress
[ ] Eating better, consulting a nutritional therapist
[ ] Seeing a doctor for your hormone issue or menopause symptoms

Environment

[ ] Stopping smoking
[ ] Avoiding the sun
[ ] Daily sunscreen

Skincare

Remember the 3 rules of skincare: keep it simple; do no harm (is your skin sensitized?); pay attention.

Have you decided on your 5 skin BASICS plus moisturizer?

[ ] Sunscreen
[ ] Cleanser
[ ] Vitamin A
[ ] Acid exfoliant
[ ] Antioxidant serum - vitamin C
[ ] Moisturizer

Do you want to start with one of the specialized skincare programmes (see pages 143-56)?

[ ] Reset for dull, dehydrated skin
[ ] Reset for mature skin
[ ] Reset for pigmentation
[ ] Intervention for sensitized skin
[ ] Intervention for rosacea
[ ] Intervention for adult acne

Skinscore

Look back at your skin concerns on page 169.

Here's another opportunity to work out yours. Which of the signs of ageing has got the highest score, and therefore is most important to you?

	Score (0–3)	Concern? (0–3)
DULL, DEHYDRATED		
REDNESS		
PIGMENTATION		
WRINKLES		
CRÊPINESS		
LOSS OF FIRMNESS		
VOLUME LOSS		

What skincare, maintenance, regeneration or optimizing treatments have you noted down to treat this concern?

How often is it recommended that you have this treatment? How often can you have it?

My annual PAP

What do you want to put into your annual plan? Under these headings, write 1 to 3 things you'll work on in each area. Nothing is compulsory, so of course you can have none in one box, too. You can't do everything.

Ask yourself: where do I want to invest my time and money? What is most important to me?

MINDSET	
STRESS	

NUTRITION	
HORMONES	
ENVIRONMENT	
SKINCARE	
MAINTENANCE	
REGENERATION	
OPTIMIZATION	

The ages of beauty

I have mentioned ages throughout the book, to give you an idea of when you might see particular changes or benefit from particular skincare or treatment. While I think lumping advice into categories based on decades is far too general, I am always, always being asked the question, 'When should I . . . ?' in relation to various treatments, so I will try to answer that here.

Frustrating as this will be to hear if you are, say, 50, in fact all 5 forms of ageing can be minimized by starting looking after your skin in your 30s. But you can start now: the more proactive and not reactive you can be at any age, the better the results.

If I had to put an age on it, I would say there are transition points, when people notice their skin has changed. These are the most frequent ages of first visit to the clinic: 35, 42, 49, 55. But please be aware, your transition point could be a few years before or after this. It all depends on your genetics, plus lifestyle, plus life stage, plus how you've cared for your skin. The following advice is based on these transition points but, because of your individual factors, it might not suit you exactly, so please treat it as a very rough guide.

Advice for all ages

Sun, sugar, smoking - stop now! At the very least, cut down. The same goes for negative self-talk. If you find it hard to do this for yourself, think about your daughter, niece, granddaughter or goddaughter. If you can stop it, you won't pass the habit on to the younger generation.

Caitlin Moran says this, in *More Than a Woman*:

'And whatever you choose to do, it's important to remember the biggest, and most crucial thing about ageing: every so often, you will look at pictures of yourself from ten years ago - when you were convinced you looked shit and were going downhill - and exclaim: "My God - I was so young and hot back then! I was at my *peak*! Look at my fucking *legs*! They're like those of a *sexy horse*! Why did I not *appreciate* it at the time? I should have just walked around *naked* all the time insisting people take pictures of my face! I will never be that beautiful *again*!"

And this will happen every ten years until you die.'

30 to 37

This is what I call the 'driver' period, when women first become concerned about the changes in their skin, so they want to learn more. They want to know the next steps. Perhaps your usual moisturizer isn't giving the same glow, perhaps you develop a few fine lines (usually crows' feet or forehead lines). Or perhaps you're fed up with being asked if you're OK because of your furrowed brow making you look tired or stressed.

DIET: Lots of fruit and veg, nutrient-rich dishes, cooked from scratch with no processed foods.
SLEEP: Don't scrimp on sleep to fit it all in, just because you feel energized and your skin is smooth . . . for now! Start your own #sleeprevolution.
EXERCISE: Move! Regularly. But you know that.
STRESS MANAGEMENT: Keep your stress down with the advice that starts on page 55. If you can establish daily stress-fighting habits, so much the better. It's just as important to focus on stress as it is to exercise regularly and sleep and eat well. Lay the foundations, you WILL reap the benefits in the years to come.
SKIN CANCER CHECK: Start having an annual one now.
SKINCARE: Find your 5 basics. Wear sunscreen every day. Cleanse twice per day. Use a leave-on acid exfoliant for glow. Vitamin A is your best investment. If you do want a serum, Vitamin C is excellent.
MAINTENANCE: 6+ facials a year including acid exfoliant peels will help give you stand-out skin. Monthly facials and/or mesotherapy and/or IPL and/or microneedling if you want to step it up.

37 to 45

Typically, the women I see in this age bracket are frazzled. They are burning the candle at 3 ends: children, working and running a home. Pregnancy, motherhood and bad sun habits from 20 years ago are starting to show too. Age 42 is often what people call the 'dipping point', appearance-wise. Women report dull skin, redness, pigmentation as well as wrinkles and some early volume loss - all topped off with spots, too, which people don't talk about enough. It is totally *normal.* Inflamm-ageing can really kick in at this age. But you can keep it under control with:

DIET: Now is the time to consider supplements, especially if you aren't eating brilliantly (you should be!). The essentials are: omega-3 and vitamin D3+K2.

SLEEP: It's so hard not to ignore this one – sometimes it will simply be impossible, I know. But never give up, take it one day (and night) at a time, and keep it a priority.
EXERCISE: This is especially important, but needs to be something you enjoy, not another stress . . . Then you will get the psychological benefit as well as the stress-busting and all the other great benefits.
STRESS MANAGEMENT: Have some time for yourself. Somehow! Remember that phrase about putting on your oxygen mask first? It's true!
SKINCARE: Consider a reset programme. Pick the one that suits your skin issue (see page 144).
FACIALS: Maintenance facials. These make a big difference now. Ideally a monthly facial. But if you don't have the means or the time, up your exfoliation at home and use a prescription retinoid (if not pregnant or breastfeeding).
LASER: Even out skin tone. This will give you the option to wear less make-up. Laser for red vessels around the nose twice per year; IPL for pigmentation every autumn.
BTX AND FILLERS: This can tweak your blink impression. BTX for frown and crows' feet. 1 to 4 syringes of filler with a maintenance visit once per year to lift cheek contours and/or optimize proportions.

45 to 50

New beginnings! Right now, perhaps the kids are no longer so physically demanding. And you might be at the top of your game at work. But you are also experiencing perimenopause, ageing parents, the ups and downs of a longer relationship. And possibly a bit more space to think, take stock . . . and have a mid-life crisis.

HORMONES: Find the right people to advise you about menopause, sooner rather than later. Your first stop will be your GP, although not all GPs are in favour of HRT, if that is what you decide. The other options are a gynaecologist, a functional medicine practitioner, or a specialist menopause clinic. You may also want to see a nutritionist for a tailored food plan.

EXERCISE: Aim for a minimum 30 minutes of activity per day. A brisk walk is better than nothing. But a workout that uses bodyweight, such as yoga or Pilates and/or weights, is even better, to boost your muscle strength and bone density. Add a supplement to support your bones that contains both calcium and vitamin D.

NUTRITION: The power of food to reverse faulty repair and renewal processes and support hormonal imbalance is enormous. Plan your meals following all the advice from pages 84–91.

SKINCARE: Dryness from reduced sebum and increased moisture loss starts to become an issue. Invest in two cleansers: try a cream/balm/oil cleanser for every day, then an acid cleanser 2 to 3 times per week. Vitamin A is a must; prioritize this over stepping-up exfoliation. Antioxidants are important both for supporting repair and boosting defence, alongside essential daily sunscreen. Using an HA mist/serum immediately before moisturizing will also help.

SKIN BOOSTERS: Or, as I call it, 'injectable moisturizer' - twice per year will make a difference to the quality of your skin.

SKIN-TIGHTENING: You'll get a big benefit from skin-tightening: that might be from microneedling, radio-frequency or ultrasound EBDs. Maintenance facials are still very important, but even better when combined with these regenerative treatments.

FILLERS: Choose fillers over BTX. A combination of the two is best, but volume loss is more ageing than wrinkles now.

50 to 59

At last, a more balanced state of mind and wellbeing, hopefully with stress management on its way to being mastered. But looking in the mirror? It just may not look like you. Low oestrogen shows up on your skin: wrinkles and shadows deepen, and all you see is sag. Body changes are a huge impetus to come to the clinic too, from fat pockets to skin laxity. This is when you'll get the biggest benefit from doing the whole of the PAP, top to bottom. In particular, try to get rid of the habit of using sugar to rev yourself up, or wine to wind down.

HORMONES: Everything comes back to them. If you feel tired or sad or angry, it may be your hormones. See your GP if you haven't already.
BREAST CHECK: Mammograms are available through the NHS every 3 years from 50+.
EXERCISE: Keep it up. The key to this is doing something you love, so that you look forward to it rather than dreading it.
SKINCARE: The same advice applies as on page 259, but you might also need a richer moisturizer to use at night. Facial oils are a great add-on - go for 100% plant-based. Jojoba and squalene are lighter oils, less likely to contribute to congestion.
MAINTENANCE PLUS: A comprehensive approach/annual programme including facials every 4 to 6 weeks, and incorporating regenerative treatments such as needling, PRP, Profhilo plus radio-frequency. Annual Ultherapy (see page 213) for tightening.
BTX AND FILLERS: 2 to 3 visits per year for maintenance.
LASER: Annual laser for veins, pigmentation, resurfacing as required.

60+:

Hopefully you'll have more time to yourself by now - although I know a lot of women who step up their careers at this point, as well as other commitments, so have even less. I'm sure that by now you are confident in your own identity and aware of what works for you and what makes you happy. When it comes to style, I think less make-up looks so elegant at this age. I've seen how treatments can really help women to feel groomed and together without having to turn to their old cover-ups. But the watchword is, less is more. Embracing how you look now is to embrace the essence of you and everything that has happened in your life. That is the definition of true beauty. You don't want to erase them from your life - so don't erase them from your face.

SKINCARE: As on page 259. Also, even skin tone can make an enormous difference at this age. Prescription skincare that targets brown spots, maintained by a high-quality pigmentation serum, is worth the investment. You may also want to have a laser treatment for burst blood vessels. The right skincare and monthly maintenance facials are still very important. But regenerative treatments will not be as effective - your skin won't respond in the same way. There will have been a cumulative benefit, though, if you had them when younger, and that investment will pay off.

BTX AND FILLERS: If you want to go down this route, these can still make a big difference - I tend to use far lower doses of BTX, and more filler at this age. And it really does need 'blending' all over the face for best results. Note that this will require a much higher budget, as you're looking at 8+ syringes, repeated annually. These clients usually are the ones who have actively said no to surgery because they don't want to do anything irreversible or they are mindful of the risks.

The ultimate PAP team!

If you have the time and money, and would like a truly multidisciplinary approach to positive ageing, this is the team you want on your side. This may sound expensive but there are lots of DIY and group options now. Joining in is a great way to motivate yourself and sustain behavioural change. You can also have online consultations, or find an expert whose approach you like and follow them online. (Do check expert qualifications. And if you have any health conditions, ask your GP.)

- Functional medicine practitioner(s) - this may include a doctor, nutritional therapist and/or a health coach
- Aesthetician (skincare, facials)
- Aesthetic doctor (regenerative and corrective treatments)
- Dermatologist (skin check/skin disease)
- Gynaecologist/GP (HRT, smear, mammograms)

- Support team of PT, hairdresser, dental hygienist, make-up – LIGHTS, CAMERA, ACTION!

What are your daily priorities?

This is it. This is where the magic lies. Because what you do every day is what you will become. Now you've decided how you're going to build your annual plan from the PAP, work back in order to plan your daily priorities – starting tomorrow.

I've given an example of mine below. Mine is personal to me. I have three school-age children and I have to prioritize sleep or I can't function at work or home. Each week, I look at my list of priorities and work out how and when I'm going to achieve them each day (and sometimes if!). Some take practically no time, so are non-negotiables, such as my supplements and skincare. I call them priorities rather than a to-do list because, while I aim to do them all, I don't beat myself up if I don't tick them off.

Enjoy taking these first steps into positive ageing. Listen to your body and skin at each stage to get the most out of everything you've learned. Keep looking at your list and updating it – these won't be your forever priorities. I revisit mine every few weeks or so. And be confident that you are doing what is best for your skin – but for your health, too.

- 20 minutes of morning yoga.
- My boys. Maxi, Lysander, Theo and Geoff. One-on-one time.
- 7 hours' sleep (at least!). Go to bed at 10 p.m.
- Plant-based diet, lots of variety, cooked from scratch.
- Exercise 5 days per week (I try!). That might be boxing, weights, Pilates or power yoga, or a 5k park run/walk with my headphones on.
- Daily supplements. Prescribed by HumanPeople.com, personalized daily packs tweaked every 3 months.

- My morning and evening skincare routine.
- Time alone. To read, listen to music, just be.
- A moment of connection or community. My sister, brothers, my parents, my friends.
- Time spent working on (not just in) my business – my dreams!

Now, it's your turn . . .

Here are my top 7 pieces of advice for you to always keep in mind as you go forward on your positive ageing journey. Remind yourself of these if you're ever wondering whether you're going in the right direction, or if you lose sight of your goals. You've got this!

1. Know that lifestyle change takes effort. In fact, research from University College London has shown that it takes an average of 66 days for a new behaviour to become automatic, with individual times varying from 18 to a whopping 254 days! Changing your lifestyle will take a lot more of your own willpower and regular input than putting yourself into the hands of a doctor in a clinic, but it's also free and often makes the biggest difference by far.
2. Starting at the bottom reaps results. As I've said, you can jump in at the top of the PAP pyramid but you really see more benefits when you focus on mindset and lifestyle too. If you can only do one thing today, do something to reduce your stress.
3. Zoom out. Try to take your whole face into consideration, your blink impression. Try not to focus on the things you don't like, the flaws. If you asked a friend – or me – they would likely say they haven't even noticed what you see as a flaw.
4. Even once you've set up your self-care as a personalized annual programme, you can review it regularly. But be consistent: remember that the habit you've discarded is spending time and money switching between a lot of poorly

thought-out SOS quick fixes. Aesthetic treatments are so often seen as a quick fix or cheating, but I hope I've shown you that this doesn't work.

5. You need to wait for results. A true skin upgrade, both structural and functional, that will last more than 5 days, needs at least 12 weeks to kick in before it becomes visible and sustainable. It will be worth that wait.
6. Do what you can. Be proud of yourself for looking after yourself, whatever you do. You can't do everything! Even the clients I see whose looks are their career have to prioritize according to time and money.
7. Finally, stay positive. Think little and often. Positive ageing is all about forming positive habits. Our attitude to ageing in the past was always that we were 'anti', to fight it at all costs. Let's embrace ageing, but do it our way. Let's use the advances of science to ensure we are happy when we look in the mirror but know that, underneath, how we are living is good for our health, too.

Positive ageing means knowing we are at our most beautiful, no matter what other people think. It's about feeling good in our skin, and our skin being in its best and glowiest condition. How you choose to present yourself to the world is your business. My wish is that this book gives you the exact tools to do that.

Skincare programmes

The Reset for dull and dehydrated skin

WEEKS	A.M.	P.M. (DAY 1)	P.M. (DAY 2)	P.M. (DAY 3)
Stage 1: STRIP BACK [Weeks 1 and 2]				
1, 2	Cleanse Moisturize Sunscreen	Cleanse Moisturize		
Stage 2: TREAT [Weeks 3 to 12]				
3, 4, 5	Cleanse Moisturize Sunscreen	Cleanse Acid exfoliant Moisturize		
6, 7, 8	Cleanse Antioxidant serum Moisturize Sunscreen	Cleanse Acid exfoliant Moisturize		
9, 10, 11, 12	Cleanse Antioxidant serum Moisturize Sunscreen	Cleanse Acid exfoliant Moisturize	Cleanse Vitamin A Moisturize	Cleanse Moisturize
Stage 3: MAINTAIN [Weeks 13+]				
13+	Cleanse Antioxidant serum ADD-ONS Moisturize Sunscreen	Cleanse Acid exfoliant Moisturize	Cleanse Vitamin A Moisturize	Cleanse ADD-ONS/ oils Moisturize

NOTES
Calm and support your skin barrier
Find a sunscreen you are happy using every single day, rain or shine
Introduce the 3 'A's, one at a time
Leave on exfoliant lotion/toner
Boosting defence against the environment (UV, pollution)
Rotate with acid exfoliant as tolerated. Otherwise omit the exfoliant for 3 weeks, then re-introduce
Add in targeted ingredients, one at a time, always paying attention
Add on as tolerated. Niacinamide or hyaluronic acid for a hydration boost, or potentially switching up to an exfoliating cleanser twice a week

The Reset for mature skin

WEEKS	A.M.	P.M. (DAY 1)	P.M. (DAY 2)	P.M. (DAY 3)
Stage 1: STRIP BACK [Weeks 1 and 2]				
1, 2	Cleanse Moisturize Sunscreen	Cleanse Moisturize		
Stage 2: TREAT [Weeks 3 to 12]				
3, 4, 5	Cleanse Moisturize Sunscreen	Cleanse Acid exfoliant* Moisturize	Cleanse Acid exfoliant Moisturize	Cleanse Moisturize
6, 7, 8	Cleanse Antioxidant Serum Moisturize Sunscreen	Cleanse Acid exfoliant Moisturize		
9, 10	Cleanse Antioxidant serum Moisturize Sunscreen	Cleanse Acid exfoliant Moisturize	Cleanse Vitamin A Moisturize	Cleanse Moisturize
11, 12	Cleanse Antioxidant serum Moisturize Sunscreen	Cleanse Vitamin A Moisturize	Cleanse (acid exfoliant)* Moisturize	Cleanse Vitamin A Moisturize

NOTES
Calm and support the skin barrier
Perhaps try an oil cleanser/balm cleanser
Vitamin A is key to this programme.
Start with 2 days on, 1 day off. Gradually building up to every night
Add in an antioxidant
Use the 3-2-1-Go method to introduce
Alternate day vitamin A for 2 weeks (NOT on a 3-day cycle for these 2 weeks) * Use acid exfoliant only if tolerated. If your skin is irritated, leave this step out for now.
CONT.

Stage 3: Maintenance [Weeks 13+]				
13+	Cleanse Antioxidant serum ADD-ONS Moisturize Sunscreen	Cleanse Vitamin A Moisturize	Cleanse Vitamin A/ Acid exfoliant** Moisturize	Cleanse ADD-ONS/ oils Moisturize
Harder hitting version of weeks 13+ – if using Rx tretinoin	Cleanse Antioxidant serum Moisturize Sunscreen	Cleanse Vitamin A Moisturize	Cleanse Vitamin A Moisturize	Cleanse Vitamin A Moisturize

The Reset for pigmentation

WEEKS	A.M.	P.M. (DAY 1)	P.M. (DAY 2)	P.M. (DAY 3)
Stage 1: Strip back [Weeks 1–2]				
1, 2	Cleanse Moisturize Sunscreen	Cleanse Moisturize		
Stage 2: Treat – depigmentation system [Weeks 3 to 12]				
3, 4, 5	Cleanse Acid exfoliant HQ4% (Rx only) Moisturize Sunscreen	Cleanse HQ4% (Rx only) Moisturize		

Step up to daily Vitamin A
All 5 add-ons will likely be appropriate. But keep it simple!
A good regime combined with regular maintenance facials (see Chapter 6) and/or regenerative procedures (see Chapter 7)

NOTES

Strengthening the barrier in preparation
Ceramides are good for barrier support

Triple therapy
Take both actives to hairline and as far as the orbit bone - not to neck initially

CONT.

6-12	Cleanse Antioxidant serum Acid exfoliant HQ4% (Rx only) Moisturize Sunscreen	Cleanse HQ4% (Rx only) Vitamin A (tretinoin* Rx only) Moisturize			
Stage 3: Maintenance [Months 4+]					
Months 4-8 inclusive	Cleanse Antioxidant serum/ ADD-ONS (Acid exfoliant 2-3 times a week) Moisturize Sunscreen	Cleanse Vitamin A Moisturize			
8 months+	Cleanse Antioxidant serum ADD-ONS Moisturize Sunscreen	Cleanse Acid exfoliant Moisturize	Cleanse Vitamin A Moisturize	Cleanse ADD-ONS/ oils Moisturize	

	* Starting with a pea-sized amount, building up
	Note: Continue to use Vitamin A
	Do NOT stop HQ4% abruptly (wean off over 1 month to prevent rebound hyperpigmentation)
	Pull back to using Vitamin A every 3 nights

The Intervention for all sensitized skin

*Acne and rosacea really do need to be treated in clinic - and usually combining prescription skincare with procedures (e.g. peels and laser). But here is a plan that may be useful for less aggressive flare-ups.

Add-ons such as azelaic acid and niacinamide may be introduced within this 6-week period, to help soothe.

WEEKS	A.M.	P.M. (DAY 1)	P.M. (DAY 2)	P.M. (DAY 3)
Step 1: Strip back [Weeks 1-6*]				
1-6	Cleanse Moisturize Sunscreen	Cleanse Moisturize		
Step 2: Treat [Weeks 7 onwards]				
7, 8, 9	Cleanse Moisturize Sunscreen	Cleanse Acid exfoliant Moisturize		
10, 11, 12	Cleanse Antioxidant serum Moisturize Sunscreen	Cleanse Acid exfoliant Moisturize		
Step 3: Maintenance [Weeks 13+]				
13+	Cleanse Antioxidant serum/ ADD-ONS Moisturize Sunscreen	Cleanse Acid exfoliant Moisturize	Cleanse ADD ONS Moisturize	Cleanse ADD ONS Moisturize

NOTES
Calm and repair barrier
Avoid fragrances, scrubs, hot showers
Calm, repair and boost barrier function
Salicylic acid (build up gradually to daily use)
Supporting defence and repair
Cautiously adding in one product at a time
Niacinamide, azelaic acid HA

Glossary

Acid mantle: A protective film on the surface of your skin, formed of sebum and sweat.

Advanced glycation end products (AGEs): Proteins (e.g. collagen) or lipids that become altered or 'glycated' after exposure to sugars.

Alpha hydroxy acid (AHA), e.g. glycolic, lactic acid: Chemicals that exfoliate, i.e. remove the outer layers of the epidermis. Used in skincare (cleansers, toners, pads, lotions and masks), and at stronger concentration as in-clinic treatments (peels).

Antioxidant: Protective molecules produced in the body and found in foods that help defend your cells from damage caused by potentially harmful free radicals.

Astaxanthin: A powerful antioxidant (a carotenoid) most commonly found in salmon, giving the fish its pinkish colour.

Azelaic acid: A naturally occurring acid that exfoliates but also has anti-inflammatory, anti-bacterial, anti-comedonal and antioxidant properties. An effective ingredient in acne and rosacea management.

Bakuchiol: A plant-derived antioxidant with similar benefits to vitamin A, but without the irritation or instability.

Beta hydroxy acid (BHA), e.g. salicylic acid: Fat-soluble, unlike water-soluble AHAs, and therefore better at dissolving through oils and decongesting oily, acne-prone skin. Also anti-inflammatory.

Collagen: A protein that gives skin structure - plumpness.

Cosmeceutical: A made-up word used by marketeers to elevate a product from 'purely cosmetic'. But this is a non-regulated word, so neither function nor promised benefits are guaranteed.

Cryotherapy: 'Cold therapy' is used to treat a variety of issues - originally to treat skin cancer, but now being used at different intensities within facials and for fat removal (e.g. CoolSculpting).

Dermaplaning: A skin treatment that uses an exfoliating blade to skim dead skin cells and fine hair from your face.

Dermis: The middle layer that makes up 90% of your skin. Where all your collagen and elastin fibres are, as well as blood vessels.

Elastin: The protein that gives skin its elasticity, its bounce.

Emollient: A moisturizing ingredient that smooths and softens skin.

Epidermis:The outer layer of skin, which includes the stratum corneum, the outermost layer of the epidermis. The health of your epidermis determines the strength of your skin barrier - essential for calm, clear, hydrated skin.

Exfoliation (or 'desquamation'): A natural process of cell turnover: dead cells of the stratum corneum are removed, revealing the brighter, fresher cells below. This can be accelerated by the use of chemical exfoliants (e.g. lactic acid) or physical exfoliants (mechanical scrubs).

Fibroblasts: Cells in the dermis that produce collagen and elastin fibres.

Free radicals: Highly reactive, unstable substances that can cause chain reactions leading to damage of DNA, proteins and lipids.

Gen-V facial: A fractional non-ablative laser used for skin rejuvenation. Immediately visible benefits that can include pore refinement, less redness, more plump and lift. But also some longer-lasting regenerative benefits from the stimulation of new collagen production.

Glycerin: A natural moisturizer, made by skin but also a key humectant component of many moisturizers.

Glycolic acid: A type of AHA found in sugarcane extract, considered by many to be the most effective AHA. It hydrates as well as improving radiance and evenness of tone.

Gluconolactone: An antioxidant PHA (polyhydroxyacid). A chemical exfoliant which works well for more sensitive skins.

Glycosaminoglycans (GAGs): The matrix support structure for collagen and elastin in the dermis that binds moisture. Hyaluronic acid is an important GAG.

Humectant: A moisturizing ingredient that attracts water, slowing evaporation. Occurs naturally in the body and is also a skincare ingredient.

Hyaluronic acid (HA): A humectant (skin hydration boosting molecule) found in the dermis and epidermis and important for healing and repair.

Hydroquinone: The gold standard pigment-buster. Commonly thought of as a bleaching ingredient, but actually an enzyme-blocker - blocking an enzyme that is required for cells to produce new brown pigment (melanin). Requires a prescription at higher strengths (4% in the UK).

INCI: International Nomenclature of Cosmetic Ingredients, i.e. the list of product ingredients.

IPL (intense pulsed light): A treatment that uses high-energy beams of light, pushed into the face via a handpiece to improve your skin tone. It reduces red and brown pigment to make your complexion more even.

Juvederm: A leading brand of injectable filler with a base of hyaluronic acid.

Keratinocyte: An epidermal cell - the 'bricks' of its brick and mortar structure - that produces keratin. This is the same tough protein that is found in hair and nails.

Lactic acid: A gentle alpha hydroxy acid - a chemical exfoliant.

Langerhans cells: Immune cells of the epidermis.

Lipids: Or 'oils' in skincare. Substances that don't dissolve in water (triglycerides, fatty acids, ceramides and cholesterol).

Matrix metalloproteinases (MMPs): Enzymes that can break down structural proteins in skin, such as collagen. Photo-aged skin has a high level of MMPs.

Melanin: The pigment that gives skin, eyes and hair their colour. It protects by absorbing UVB energy.

Melanocytes: Cells that produce melanin.

Mesotherapy: The 'vitamin facial': a combination of very light needling while simultaneously introducing ingredients (a mix of vitamins, minerals, antioxidants and hyaluronic acid) deeper than if they are applied locally. To tighten and brighten skin.

Microbiome: All the microbes - bacteria, fungi and viruses - that live on and inside the human body.

Microneedling: 'Dermaroller' is a well-known brand name. A treatment in which thousands of tiny, controlled wounds are created in the skin by multiple, tiny needles (up to 3mm long). Can be used lightly to simply improve penetration of products used immediately after, or deeply to trigger a 'wound healing' response, stimulating the skin to produce new collagen and elastin. This can help with acne scarring, stretch marks and pigmentation, as well as being an excellent treatment for all-round rejuvenation.

Niacinamide: Vitamin B3. Boosts ceramide production and so supports our skin barrier. Also great for redness and breakouts (anti-inflammatory), pigmentation and wrinkles.

Occlusive: Moisturizes by adding a layer that seals. Can exacerbate congestion.

OTC (over the counter): No prescription needed.

Peptide: Protein 'cell messengers' that can influence skin function at a cellular level.

PHA (polyhydroxy acid): A special 'next generation' type of AHA that allows for more gradual penetration and absorption and so is non-irritating.

Pigmentation: A shorthand version of 'hyperpigmentation', the darkened colouring of skin often triggered by external factors (e.g. sun, trauma, pollution, spots).

PIH: Post-inflammatory hyperpigmentation, usually caused by damage to the skin, e.g. a peel or laser treatment.

Profhilo: An extremely popular 'skin booster' regenerative treatment. Injectable hyaluronic acid that does not 'fill' but rather boosts hydration and elasticity, as well as new collagen production.

PRP, aka 'The Vampire Facial': Platelet-rich plasma. A treatment that involves taking a small amount of blood from a vein in your arm. It's spun in a centrifuge to separate out the part of the blood that's rich in platelets and so in growth factors. This is then injected into your skin to boost skin repair and function.

Radio-frequency (RF): Regenerative, skin-tightening treatments which use heat to trigger new collagen and elastin production and improve skin firmness.

Retinoids: An umbrella term for vitamin A derivatives, e.g. retinol, tretinoin.

Sebum: Natural moisturizing lipids produced by skin's sebaceous glands – flows on to the surface through pores.

Stratum corneum: Dead but important outermost layer of the epidermis.

References

Cao, C., Xiao, Z., Wu, Y. and Ge, C. (2020), 'Diet and Skin Aging - From the Perspective of Food Nutrition', *Nutrients*, 12 (3), p. 870.

Ehlinger-Martin, A., Cohen-Letessier, A., Taïeb, M., Azoulay, E. and du Crest, D. (2015), 'Women's attitudes to beauty, aging, and the place of cosmetic procedures: insights from the QUEST Observatory', *Journal of Cosmetic Dermatology*, 15 (1), pp. 89–94.

Fabbrocini, G., Bertona, M., Picazo, Ó., Pareja-Galeano, H., Monfrecola, G. and Emanuele, E. (2016), 'Supplementation with Lactobacillus rhamnosus SP1 normalises skin expression of genes implicated in insulin signalling and improves adult acne', *Beneficial Microbes*, 7 (5), pp. 625–30.

Galvão Cândido, F., Xavier Valente, F., da Silva, L.E., Gonçalves Leão Coelho, O., Gouveia Peluzio, M. do C. and Gonçalves Alfenas, R. de C. (2017), 'Consumption of extra virgin olive oil improves body composition and blood pressure in women with excess body fat: a randomized, double-blinded, placebo-controlled clinical trial', *European Journal of Nutrition*, 57 (7), pp. 2445–55.

J, H.-L., Tb, S., M, B., T, H. and D, S. (2015), 'Loneliness and Social Isolation as Risk Factors for Mortality: A Meta-Analytic Review', [online] *Perspectives on psychological science : a journal of the Association for Psychological Science*. Available at: https://pubmed.ncbi.nlm.nih.gov/25910392/.

Jeong, J. H., Lee, C. Y. and Chung, D. K. (2015), 'Probiotic Lactic Acid Bacteria and Skin Health', *Critical Reviews in Food Science and Nutrition*, 56 (14), pp. 2331–7.

Krutmann, J., Moyal, D., Liu, W., Kandahari, S., Lee, G.-S., Nopadon, N., Xiang, L.F. and Seité, S. (2017), 'Pollution and acne: is there a link?' *Clinical, Cosmetic and Investigational Dermatology*, [online] 10, pp. 199–204. Available at: https://www.ncbi.nlm.nih.gov/pmc/articles/PMC5446966/.

Melov, S., Tarnopolsky, M. A., Beckman, K., Felkey, K. and Hubbard, A. (2007), 'Resistance Exercise Reverses Aging in Human Skeletal Muscle', *PLoS ONE*, [online] 2 (5), p.e465. Available at: https://www.ncbi.nlm.nih.gov/pmc/articles/PMC1866181/ [Accessed 6 Dec. 2019].

Miyazaki, K., Masuoka, N., Kano, M. and Iizuka, R. (2014), 'Bifidobacterium fermented milk and galacto-oligosaccharides lead to improved skin health by decreasing phenols production by gut microbiota', *Beneficial Microbes*, 5 (2), pp. 121–8.

Randhawa, M., Wang, S., Leyden, J. J., Cula, G. O., Pagnoni, A. and Southall, M. D. (2016), 'Daily Use of a Facial Broad Spectrum Sunscreen Over One Year Significantly Improves Clinical Evaluation of Photoaging', *Dermatologic surgery: official publication for American Society for Dermatologic Surgery [et al.]*, [online] 42 (12), pp. 1354–61. Available at: https://www.ncbi.nlm.nih.gov/pubmed/27749441 [Accessed 10 Feb. 2020].

Sherman, K. A., Roper, T. and Kilby, C. J. (2019), 'Enhancing self-compassion in individuals with visible skin conditions: randomised pilot of the "My Changed Body" self-compassion writing intervention', *Health Psychology and Behavioral Medicine*, 7 (1), pp. 62–77.

Smith, T. J., Wilson, M., Karl, J. P., Orr, J., Smith, C., Cooper, A., Heaton, K., Young, A. J. and Montain, S. J. (2018), 'Impact of sleep restriction on local immune response and skin barrier restoration with and without "multinutrient" nutrition intervention', *Journal of Applied Physiology*, 124 (1), pp. 190–200.

Stevenson, S. and Thornton, J. (2007), 'Effect of estrogens on skin aging and the potential role of SERMs', *Clinical Interventions in Aging*, [online] 2 (3), pp. 283–97. Available at: https://www.ncbi.nlm.nih.gov/pmc/articles/PMC2685269/.

Acknowledgements

Max, Lysander and Theo, thank you for keeping meticulous track of my word count and always instantly snapping me back to being present, every time I look up from my screen. With you three, I feel so much love and heart-bursting joy. You make me incredibly proud. Never a day goes by that I don't thank my lucky stars for having you boys in my life.

Geoff, thank you for your patience and encouragement. And for cooking all those weekend lunches as I plodded on! A life less ordinary, we said, and hand in hand we've chased our dreams. Much.

Mummy, for your unwavering support, unconditional love and always believing. You have selflessly given me everything I could have ever wanted. You have taught me to always show up, you give me courage. Your kindness and grit inspire me every day.

Daddy, DGD. You have pushed me to be the best I can, to always honour hard work, integrity, hope and perseverance. You are always in my head and heart; your love and guidance give me enormous confidence and strength. I'm proud to be your Likkle Tiss.

Elisa, you are the most caring and supportive sister a girl could ask for. Thank you for always being there for me, my safe space full of laughter and love.

Simon, Katie, Susi and to all my beautiful confidantes and comrades. You make my life infinitely better.

Venetia, the hugest thank you for the hundredth time for believing in me. Watch this space! Brigid, your straight-talking input was so appreciated, and thank you for taking the reins when my impetus waned, for getting this book over the line. Amy, your patience and guidance have helped enormously. Annie, your attention to detail is mindblowing, thank you! And thank you to the rest of the publishing team at Penguin Life for your support and to Elizabeth at PFD for making this happen.

Lastly to the team at Medicetics and to all my wonderful clients, who have had faith in me and embraced my guidance over the years. I have learned so much from your time 'on the chair', about aesthetics and well beyond! Helping you to feel amazing is my passion and the greatest reward. This book is for you.

Index

Page references in *italics* indicate images.

INDEX

INDEX